YOGA

Whatever your age, sex, creed or race, you can achieve the same results by following this wonderful life-science—glowing health, increased energy and stamina, a shaplier body, relaxation, improved concentration, peace of mind.

YOGA

JAMES HEWITT

HODDER PAPERBACKS

ISBN 0 340 15581 7

CONTENTS

▼

ACKNOWLEDGMENTS

I thank the following for giving permission to quote extracts:

Mr. Alain Danielou and Christopher Johnson Publishers Ltd., from *Yoga, The Method of Re-integration*; Dr. Albert Schweitzer and A. & C. Black Ltd., from *Indian Thought and Its Development* and *The Ethics of Reverence for Life*; Dr. W. Y. Evans-Wentz and Oxford University Press, from *The Tibetan Book of The Dead*; Mr. F. Yeats-Brown and Victor Gollancz Ltd., from *Yoga Explained*; Dr. Lily Abegg and Thames and Hudson Ltd., from *The Mind of East Asia*; Mr. Mouni Sadhu and George Allen & Unwin Ltd., from *In Days of Great Peace*; Dr. Innes H. Pearse and Lucy H. Crocker, B.Sc. and George Allen & Unwin Ltd., from *The Peckham Experiment*; Mr. Romain Rolland and Cassell and Co. Ltd., from *Prophets of the New India*; The Public Trustee and The Society of Authors, from George Bernard Shaw's *Man and Superman*; Mr. Romain Rolland and George G. Harrap and Co Ltd., from *Jean-Christophe*; the late Dr. Alexis Carrel and Hamish Hamilton Ltd., from *Man The Unknown*; the late Dr. Maurice Nicoll and Vincent Stuart, Publishers Ltd., from *Living Time and the Integration of the Life*; the late Theos. Bernard and Rider & Co., from *Hatha Yoga*; Dr. Paul Brunton and Rider & Co., from *The Quest of The Overself*; Mr. Aldous Huxley and Chatto and Windus Ltd., from *The Perennial Philosophy* and *Ends and Means*; Mr. George A. Dorsey and Harper and Brothers, New York, from *Why We Behave Like Humans*; the late Sri Aurobindo and the Sri Aurobindo Ashram, Pondicherry, India. Advaita Ashrama, Calcutta for extracts from Swami Vivekananda's *Raja Yoga, Bhakti Yoga* and *Practical Vedanta*.

INTRODUCTION

WHAT IS YOGA?

Self-Realization

Yoga goes back two thousand years before the birth
of Christ. The first written account of its teachings
was by the Indian Patanjali, probably in the second
century. The word 'Yoga' is derived through the
Sanskrit, from the same Indo-European root as the
English 'to yoke'. It can also be translated as 'union'
or 'identification'. This 'union' is the merging of the
individual soul with the universal soul. The Yogi
believes that there is a universal Overself with whom
he can make contact and identify himself in moments
of higher consciousness. By a programme of bodily
and mental self-discipline we who move on lower
levels of consciousness can achieve Samadhi (union
with divine consciousness). This is the moment of
spiritual illumination, of self-realization. It is the
meditative bliss of the religious mystic throughout the
ages. Poets, artists and musicians have been touched
at times by the divine breath. And we too may have
experienced it in those moments—very often in
childhood—when we were carried out of ourselves
on being confronted by the beautiful and the wonderful. Visvanatha has said: "The experience of beauty

is pure, self-manifested, compounded equally of joy and consciousness, free from admixture of any other perception, the very twin brother of mystical experience, and the very life of it is supersensuous wonder." The Yoga teaching is that all can strive for such experience, and that many paths can be taken to attain it.

In the *Yoga Sara Sangraha* we find this definition: "The silencing of the mind's activities which leads to the complete realization of the intrinsic nature of the Supreme Person is called Yoga." The *Bhagavad Gita* says: "The yogi who has conquered himself, whose inner peace is not disturbed by cold or heat, pain or pleasure, honours or insults, whose all being is set on the Supreme Self, whose inner faculties are satiated with knowledge and Transcendent Wisdom without impulses, his sense mastered, looking to mud and gold with an equal eye, is said to be yoked."

Yoga is therefore a spiritual technique, a method, a way, a path. It is not a religion, but is nevertheless a spiritual exercise or meditative technique for the religious.

The sacred writings of all the major religions advise such meditation.

Buddhism

There is no meditation apart from wisdom.
    There is no wisdom apart from meditation.
Those in whom wisdom and meditation meet
    Are not far from peace.

                                        (*Dhammapada*).

Taoism

Those whose hearts are in a state of repose
   give forth a divine radiance
      by which they see themselves as they are.
   And only by cultivating such repose
      can man attain to the constant.

(Kwang Tze).

Jainism

He who is rich in control renounces everything,
   and meditates on the reflections on life.
He whose soul is purified by meditating
   is compared to a ship in water.
Like a ship reaching the shore, he gets beyond
      misery.

(Sutra-Kritanga Sutra).

Christianity

Whatsoever things are true,
   whatsoever things are honest,
whatsoever things are just,
   whatsoever things are pure,
whatsoever things are lovely,
   whatsoever things are of good report,
if there be any virtue,
   and if there be any praise,
think on these things.

(Philippians).

Islam

Meditate on thy Lord in thine own mind with
humility
and without loud speaking, evening and morning.
And be not one of the negligent.

(Koran).

Hinduism

Whoever here among men attain greatness,
they have, as it were, part of the reward of
meditation.
Reverence meditation.

He who reverences meditation as the Supreme—
as far as meditation goes,
so far he has unlimited freedom.

(Chandogya Upanishad).

Sikhism

The world is an ocean, and difficult to cross.
How shall man traverse it?

As a lotus in the water remaineth dry,
As also a water-fowl in the stream—
So by meditating on the Word
Shalt thou be unaffected by the world.

(Guru Nanak).

The spiritual exercises of St. Ignatius of Loyola included Yoga-like practices. Buddhist meditation utilizes Yoga, especially the Yogacara school which lays emphasis on the trance. But the most detailed descriptions of Yoga methods are to be found in the sacred works of the Hindu, such as the Vedas, the Tantras, etc. "From the point of view of their ultimate significance all the Hindu scriptures, indeed the scriptures of all religions, may be said to be treatises of Yoga", writes Alain Danielou in his *Yoga: The Method of Re-Integration*. "The aim of all religions is to bring man towards union with, or re-integration into the Supreme Being. Religious practices or moral disciplines are only preliminary stages in this process."

There is nothing in Yoga that should offend people of the Christian or any other faith. Yoga teaches the unity of all life and sets out a programme of practical exercises whereby you can experience this. Anyone can benefit from Yoga. The believer who practises it will be brought closer to God. Ramakrishna says: "Through Yoga a Hindu becomes a better Hindu, a Christian a better Christian, a Mohammedan a better Mohammedan, and a Jew a better Jew."

Equally, an agnostic or atheist may practise Yoga and derive great benefit. This may seem strange until you come to understand just what the Yoga techniques involve. The system of physical mastery known as Hatha Yoga, and the system of psychical mastery known as Raja Yoga—the two Yogas with which this work is chiefly concerned—constitute in them-

The Yogi student must see for himself that he is not the body, feelings, personality, or intellect, but their user. The pure Self is concealed like the sun behind cloud. Only by the most diligent self-training can it be revealed and experienced as reality.

Bhakti involves faith and worship. It is the Yoga of devotion, involving concentration and meditation on the Divine. It is the way of the emotions as Jnana is of the intellect. It asks for service to your fellow men and complete unselfishness.

Karma is for the active and the extravert. It is work performed for the service of mankind, and at the same time it is worship. The craftsman worships with his tools, the farmer with his plough.

Vivekananda believed in a synthesis of the various Yogas—Jnana, Bhakti, Karma, Raja—to achieve self-realization. And he warned against life-negation. Meditation should not lead to introspective egoism, but to an annihilation of egoism and the feeling of identification with all people, in whom one recognizes one's own Self. Thus the Yogi should seek to serve others. Not "I", but "Thou", said Vivekananda, should be the watchword of all well-being. "Here is the world and it is full of misery. Go out into it as Buddha did and struggle to lessen it or die in the attempt. Forget yourselves; this is the first lesson to be learnt, whether you are a theist or an atheist, whether you are an agnostic or a Vedantist, a Christian or a Mohammedan." (*Practical Vedanta*).

Mantra concentrates the mind by means of Japa,

the repetition of prayers and incantations. The Japa may be voiced, whispered, or mental. Mantra deals with the subject of sound vibrations, and there is much in this path that will fascinate the musician.

Hatha enables you to understand your body and gain mastery over it.

It is Hatha Yoga which makes the most immediate appeal to the Occidental, and it is this Yoga that is best known in the West. Physical exercises, hygiene, breathing practices, etc., are all part of Hatha Yoga. The ancient Yogis had an astounding knowledge of the workings of the human body. It was this knowledge—together with the study of the stretching movements of jungle animals (especially those of the cat family)—that enabled them to formulate the most perfect of all systems for achieving and maintaining bodily health and fitness. The superiority of this system over others lies in the fact that it aims at developing not just muscular strength or size, but the health and efficiency of the internal organs: the heart, lungs, glands, nerves, and so on. Also, it does not require any apparatus and can be practised in a confined space.

Raja Yoga is closely linked with the Hatha and they are often practised together. Some Yogi authorities lay great stress on the bodily Hatha Yoga, while others of the Raja Yoga school consider only a little Hatha necessary and rely entirely on psychic development. Just as the Hatha aims at mastering the body, so Raja aims at mastering the mind. It seeks to gain control over the stream of thoughts that flow through the human mind. It seeks to check that flow and still the mind by means of Concentration (Dharana) and Contemplation (Dhyana). By these practices a state of Superconsciousness (Samadhi) may be achieved.

Just as Everest could not have been conquered by weaklings, so the Yogi knows that to reach his spiritual goal his body must be at its fittest and most efficient and the mind must be conquered and made the servant of the Self.

Hatha and Raja Yoga are therefore means to an end, but even if you ignore the end and think only of the means, you have on the one hand the world's finest physical-culture system, and on the other hand a method of mental mastery that puts expensive mind-training courses in the shade.

Romain Rolland, in *Prophets of the New India*, says: "Normally we waste our energies. Not only are they squandered in all directions by the tornado of exterior impressions; but even when we manage to shut doors and windows, we find chaos within ourselves, a multitude like the one that greeted Julius Caesar in the Roman Forum; thousands of unexpectedly and mostly 'undesirable' guests invade and trouble us. No inner activity can be seriously effective and continuous until we have first reduced our house to order, and then have recalled and reassembled our herd of scattered energies."

Raja Yoga is designed to do just that—put our mental house in order and concentrate our scattered energies. It integrates the mind, stills its turbulence, cleanses it, strengthens it. Just as a body that has been cleansed of its toxic waste becomes healthier and stronger, so a mind emptied of its encumbering dross becomes healthier and stronger. Regular Raja Yoga practice builds up a store of mental energy that will remain on tap.

By holding the mind steady in Dharana dormant powers are awakened. Some readers may question this, but Yoga students testify that it is so. Those familiar with the psychology of the subconscious will understand the seeming paradox that when the mind is relaxed and held steady in a receptive state many creative and intellectual problems will work themselves out to a solution, magically and effortlessly. As a writer, I experience this regularly.

Laya (Latent) Yoga is a combination of many Yogas—breathing, postures, listening to inner sounds, etc., including the mysterious *Kundalini* Yoga. This sets out to awaken what is symbolically described as Kundalini, "the coiled serpent" said to sleep at the base of the spine, which when aroused travels upwards through the sushumna or spinal channel, passing through various centres or chakras until, when it reaches the centre of consciousness in the brain, a superconscious state is achieved. There is a considerable literature on the symbology of the chakras, depicted in ancient Yogi literature as a series of many-petalled flowers, bearing numerous symbols. Some modern investigators approximate the chakras with the principal nerve ganglia, others with the glands. It is a Yoga fraught with danger for those who would tamper with it without the guidance of a qualified teacher.

Yoga Miracles. Live Burial, Acid Drinking.

Many people mentally associate Yoga with such feats as being buried alive, drinking acid, or lying on a bed of nails. The genuine Yogi deplores such exhibitionism. The limb withering fakir, the bed of nails and the hair shirt are perversions of Yoga. The Sanskrit text-books clearly state that excessive asceticism is not necessary. Moderation is to be the rule. In the *Bhagavad Gita* we find this advice:

"O white Arjuna, this yoga is not attained by him who eats too much, nor by him who abstains from food. Nor by him who oversleeps nor him who keeps awake.

"This yoga which destroys pain is achieved by him who eats and behaves as is proper, whose all actions are led by reason, whose sleep and wake are regulated."

In spite of this, sensational displays of bodily or psychic powers are quite often encountered in the East.

The burial alive of the Yogi Haridas in 1837 was authentically corroborated by Sir Claude Wade, Dr. Janos Honiberger and the British Consul at Lahore. Reports state that Haridas took only milk for several days before the burial. On the day of the burial he ate nothing, but performed the Yogic internal cleansing method of swallowing a long strip of cloth, retaining it for a while in the stomach to absorb bile, etc. Then he performed another internal cleansing exercise, nauli, standing up to his neck in warm water and washing out the colon. All the openings of his body were then stopped up with wax. As do many Yogis he had cut the root of his tongue so that it could be rolled back to seal the entrance to the throat. Haridas was wrapped in linen and placed in a box which was locked by the Maharaja of Lahore and kept in a summer house with sealed door and windows. The house was guarded day and night by the Maharaja's bodyguard. After forty days the box was opened. The Yogi's servant washed his master with warm water, removed the wax stoppers and put warm yeast on his scalp. He forced the teeth open with a knife and unfolded the tongue. Tongue and eyelids were then rubbed with butter. After half-an-hour Haridas 'came to life', seemingly none the worse for his experience.

Mr. F. Yeats-Brown, in his *Yoga Explained*, tells of a Yogi who delighted in drinking acid. "A remarkable Yogi died recently in Rangoon. His name was Narasingha Swami. In December 1934, he gave an exhibition at Calcutta University before Sir C. V. Raman and other distinguished people, during which he drank lethal doses of sulphuric acid, nitric acid, and carbolic acid, laying them first on the palm of his hand, and then licking them up with his tongue. In March 1935, he went to Rangoon, where he several times swallowed the favourite poisons of suicides, including a gramme of potassium cyanide, without any ill effects.

"He did this once too often, however. One night he went home, apparently none the worse for eating broken glass and half-inch nails, as well as drinking aqua regia, and sat talking with some visitors until midnight, omitting to cleanse his alimentary canal by passing several quarts of water in one stream from mouth to anus, as was his usual custom. Presently he complained of a stomach-ache; then his right leg became paralysed. He was removed to a hospital and died twelve hours later."

Whether one deplores their ostentatious nature or not, such feats as the two described above do show the amazing knowledge of body, mind and the laws of life possessed by the Indian Yogi.

Wisdom of the East

A certain conceit and intellectual snobbishness sometimes makes Westerners intolerant of any suggestion that a half-naked Yogi seated cross-legged in a Himalayan cave may know more in some respects than a person educated in a Western university and living in a smart home full of up to date comforts and labour saving devices. They forget that the Orientals had their civilizations long before we did and that Occidental scientists are still making discoveries that have been known to the East for thousands of years, but descriptions of which are often clothed in obscure and symbolic language.

In the West we have explored and dissected the

external world, while the Oriental thinkers and scholars have been more concerned with penetrating the inner world of consciousness. They sought the laws of the universe inside themselves, believing their consciousness to be microcosm in macrocosm. It is significant that psychology, the study of mind, is the youngest Western science.

An expert on the East, Dr. Paul Brunton, in his book *The Quest of The Overself*, says:

"We Westerners are rightly proud of our achievements in 'face-lifting' this world of ours, but we get a little disturbed sometimes when we hear of a half-naked fakir performing a feat which we can neither match nor understand. The thing keeps on occurring sufficiently often to remind us that there are ancient secrets and hoary wisdom in the lands which lie east of Suez, and that the inhabitants of these colourful countries are not all the benighted heathens some of us think they are. We picture these Yogis as dreaming enthusiasts who desert the normal ways of mankind to go off into strange hiding-places, into gloomy caves, lonely mountains and secluded forests. But they go off with a clear objective, setting themselves no less a task than the acquisition of a perfect and incredible control over the frail tenement of flesh. To attain this end they practise the hard and exacting discipline laid down in their traditions. That nowadays the public comes into contact mainly with vagabonds, impostors and idle tramps, who delude others, or themselves, into the belief that they are Yogis, does not invalidate the truth of the tradition nor the genuineness of its best exponents."

Health and Happiness in an Age of Stress

The age of Yoga, ignorance of its true nature, and the symbolistic obscurity of much of the writings on the subject, give many Westerners—moving as they do in a world of hustle and bustle—the impression that the system holds nothing for them and is all rather remote, vague and impractical. In this they make a grave mistake, for Yoga is the most practical available means of attaining health and happiness in an age of stress.

I am not one of those pessimists who believe that civilization should be destroyed and that we should return to something bordering on the cave-man stage of human development. The harnessing of the forces of nature, electricity, atomic energy, flying faster than sound, space exploration . . . these are wonderful achievements, triumphs for Man in his conquest of the universe. But sometimes he is inclined to forget that he is not a machine, but a living being. In the West millions live at such a hectic pace that they are committing slow suicide. Civilization imposes a stress and strain unknown to our grandparents. Man can only successfully meet this challenge by paying increasing attention to his physical and mental well-being.

Yoga provides an answer to the problem of the West.

When I first took up daily Yoga practice many years ago I kept a record of my reactions in a little notebook. Looking at it now, I see the following results.

Almost immediately was reported a definite increase in vitality. The vitality increased with the weeks. Stamina was greatly increased and I felt quite fresh even at the end of a busy day.

The postures (Asanas) made my muscles firmer and better shaped. I felt (and was) stronger and more supple. My posture became more upright and my physique more athletic.

My weight dropped by ten pounds in three months and my waistline was reduced one inch. The abdominal muscles became firmer and more defined. Bowel elimination became regular. Friends remarked how well I was looking. I felt more buoyant and youthful.

I found that my mind had become more tranquil and my temperament more placid. I was master of my emotions. I rarely gave way to anger, or the other negative emotions. My outlook on life became brighter and I had a greater zest for living. I lived more in the present, less in the past and future. I looked at the world and myself more objectively. My sense of awareness was heightened. Concentration was much improved and I could work more efficiently and for long stretches without experiencing mental fatigue.

I began to feel at one with—and reverent towards— all living things.

The author has talked with many people who have

taken up regular Yoga practice and the results he has achieved are similar to theirs and by no means exceptional. It is because of such benefits as these that scientists, writers, psychologists, artists, musicians, ballet-dancers, singers, sportsmen and sportswomen, indeed people in all walks of life, practise Yoga and are loud in praise of its help in achieving healthier, happier, and more efficient living.

It is not necessary to live a life of solitude to achieve results. You can take an active part in the hurly-burly of civilized life and the daily practice of Yoga will act as a protection from the numerous stresses of your environment. But best results are attained by exercising and meditating alone, and some quiet part of the home should be utilized for this purpose. The *Siva Samhita* makes it clear that it is not necessary to become a hermit to achieve success in Yoga:

"He who is contented with what he gets, who restrains his senses, being a householder, who is not absorbed in the household duties, certainly attains emancipation by the practice of Yoga. Even the lordly householders obtain success by Japa, if they perform the duties of Yoga properly. Let, therefore, a householder also exert in Yoga (his wealth and conditions of life are no obstacles in this). Living in the house amidst wife and children, but being free from attachment to them, practising Yoga in secrecy, a householder even finds marks of success (slowly crowning his efforts), and thus following this teaching of mine, he ever lives in blissful happiness."

PART ONE

HARMONIOUS HEALTH THROUGH HATHA YOGA

Asanas (Postures), various Kumbhakas (breathing exercises), and other divine means, all should be utilized in the practice of Hatha Yoga, till the fruit—Raja Yoga—is obtained.

Hatha Yoga Pradipika

I

THE PATH TO HEALTH (HATHA YOGA)

The Eight Limbs of Yoga

Patanjali, who has been called "the father of Yoga", states in his *Sutras* that there are eight limbs of Yoga: Abstinences (Yamas), Observances (Niyamas), Postures (Asanas), Breath Control (Pranayama), Sense Withdrawal (Pratyahara), Concentration (Dharana), Contemplation (Dhyana), and Self-realization (Samadhi). To these may be added the Six Purification Practices or Shat Karma.

The Five Abstinences (Yamas)

Certain moral disciplines are required of the Yogi before he can undertake its practice. Patanjali lists five: Non-violence (Ahimsa), Truthfulness (Satya), Non-stealing (Asteya), Chastity (Brahmacharya), and Non-receiving (Aparigrapha).

NON-VIOLENCE (AHIMSA) was the favourite precept of Mahatma Gandhi. Of it he said: "Ahimsa is not merely a negative state of harmlessness but it is a positive state of love, of doing good even to the evil-doer. But it does not mean meek submission to the will of the evil-doer: it means the putting of one's whole soul against his will. Working under this law of our being, it is possible for a single individual to defy the whole might of an unjust empire, to save his honour, his religion, his soul, and lay the foundation for that empire's fall or its regeneration.

"Non-violence in its dynamic condition means conscious suffering."

Wild animals become tame and are said to lick the hand of the Yogi secure in Ahimsa. Patanjali says: "Near him in whom non-violence has fully taken root, all beings renounce enmity."

TRUTHFULNESS (SATYA). The Yogi earnestly seeks Truth and must speak it always.

NON-STEALING (ASTEYA). This includes non-covetousness.

CHASTITY (BRAHMACHARYA). Includes not only refraining from sexual intercourse, but not thinking sex, not praising it, not joking about it, not looking with desire and not conversing in private. The Yogi living a chaste life is able to transmute his sexual energy into spiritual energy, stored in the brain and called Ojas Shakti. Brahmacharya is made easy by eating moderately, eating only natural, pure (Sattwic) foods, and by thought control.

NON-RECEIVING (APARIGRAPHA). "The mind of the man who receives gifts is acted on by the mind of the giver, so the receiver is likely to become degenerated. Receiving gifts is prone to destroy the independence of the mind, and make us slavish. Therefore, receive no gifts." (Vivekananda, *Raja Yoga*.)

The Five Observances (Niyamas)

The five observances or niyamas are: PURITY (SAUCHA), CONTENTMENT (SANTOSHA), AUSTERITY (TAPA), STUDY (SVADHYAYA) and WORSHIP OF GOD (ISHVARA PRANIDHANA).

PURITY (SAUCHA). This means both external and internal purity. The body should be kept clean always. The Yogi must wash every day, practise the purification processes and eat pure (Sattwic) foods. Inward purity is achieved through mastering the mind, concentrating it and meditating on the virtues.

CONTENTMENT (SANTOSHA) and peace of mind are gained when body and mind are kept pure. The Yogi should be cheerful, uncomplaining, free from desire and satisfied with simple needs.

AUSTERITY (TAPA). With the observance of austerity comes self-mastery and supra-natural powers (siddhis).

STUDY (SVADHYAYA). This includes the reading of the Scriptures and spoken repetition of sacred mantras and syllables (Japa). Inward mental repetition is superior to the voiced Japa.

WORSHIP OF GOD (ISHVARA PRANIDHANA). "Through the constant thought of Divinity, identification (samadhi) is reached." (Patanjali).

Hatha Yoga

Hatha Yoga consists of The Six Purification Practices (Shat Karma), the Postures (Asanas) and Breath Control (Pranayama), which bring body and mind into harmony and prepare the latter for the concentrating and stilling techniques of Raja Yoga (The Royal Path).

The Yoga Sanskrit texts refer to Hatha Yoga as the ladder to Raja Yoga. The *Goraksha Samhita* says: "The science of Hatha Yoga is the ladder which those climb who wish to reach the higher regions of the Royal Path (Raja Yoga)."

And the *Siva Samhita* says : " The Hatha Yoga cannot be obtained without the Raja Yoga, nor can the Raja Yoga be attained without the Hatha Yoga."

The word Hatha takes its meaning from the syllables 'Ha' (the sun) and 'tha' (the moon), just as Yoga itself means union, Hatha Yoga is a union of sun and moon. This is a symbolic term for the uniting of the positive and negative energies of the body.

Alain Danielou, in his *Yoga: The Method of Re-Integration*, explains: "The cosmic Principles which, in relation to the earth, manifest themselves in the planetary world as the sun and the moon are found in every aspect of existence. In man, they appear mainly under two forms, one in the subtle body, the other in the gross body. In the subtle body they appear as two channels along which our perceptions channel between the subtle centre at the base of the spinal cord and the centre at the summit of the head. These two channels are called Ida and Pingala. Ida, situated on the left side, corresponds to the cold aspect or the moon and Pingala, on the right side, to the warm aspect or the sun.

"In the gross body, the lunar and solar principles

correspond to the respiratory, cool and the digestive, warm, vital energies, and are called Prana and Apana. It is by co-ordinating these two most powerful vital impulses that the yogi achieves his aim."

Harmonious Health

There can be little need for me to stress the value of sound health. Numerous great minds have done so before me. For instance, Ariphon, the Sicyonian, said: "Without health, life is not life; life is lifeless." And Emerson said: "The first wealth is health."

The Yogis believe that sound health can be claimed by all men and women. Nature provides an illimitable fund of energy available to all living things. The fact that man disregards Nature's laws with such recklessness and still manages to exist shows the power of this life force. He may abuse it, mock it, turn his back on it, but it goes on fighting for him. How often have cases been given up as lost by the doctors, only to see life hold on by a tenuous thread and finally triumph.

It is this same life force—the Yogis call it Prana— that brings the tree to bloom, the blossom to fruit, that energizes the leaping lamb, that propels the gazelle. Each of us has a share in an ocean of energy.

Vivekananda puts it: "In an ocean there are huge waves, then smaller waves, and still smaller, down to little bubbles; but back of all these is the infinite ocean. The bubble is connected with the infinite ocean at one end, and the huge wave at the other end. So, one may be a gigantic man, and another a little bubble; but each is connected with that infinite ocean of energy which is the common birthright of every animal that exists. Wherever there is life, the storehouse of infinite energy is behind it."

If instead of battling against Nature man invoked her aid his achievements would be infinite.

The Perfect Home Exercise System

Of all home exercise systems Hatha Yoga is the most perfect.

It does not require any apparatus, and can be performed in a small space.

It does not demand a great expenditure of energy; it therefore suits people of all ages, and is ideal for the exhausting times in which we live.

With its gentle, refreshing nature Hatha Yoga has none of the drawbacks of more strenuous systems, which accumulate fatigue poisons in the muscles. While those who practise the Asanas regularly find their bodies becoming shapelier and their muscles firmer and stronger, Hatha Yoga aims primarily at organic health and not mere muscular development. Actually Yoga Asanas are postures to be held and not exercises in the normal meaning of the word. And their stretching action has a relaxing effect; a valuable asset in an age of stress.

Almost all the Asanas have a stretching action on the spine, which houses and protects the vital nerve channels. Bodily efficiency depends on each of the billions of cells making up our bodies playing its full part in the community . . . in a word, on harmony. This harmony depends more than anything else on the work of the nervous system. With the brain as the co-ordinating centre, messages pour in by means of billions of nerve fibres. Messages received by the senses are flashed to the brain where they are stored or computed and an immediate answer given. There are cells carrying nourishment, cells busy with the task of removing waste products, cells carrying messages. The nervous system is the telephone service of the cell community. Its telephone network reaches every part of our bodies.

The fine nerves coming from the sense organs group together into cables on the way to the brain exchange, the biggest cable being the spinal cord which is located in and protected by the spinal column. The importance of keeping the spine flexible and in healthy condition is obvious.

One set of nerves—the sensory—make their way with their messages to the brain, and another reaches out with the reply from the brain—the motor nerves. The brain has its own centre for distributing the work. The centre dealing with sight, for example, is to the rear of the cerebrum, the centre for hearing just below the Fissure of Sylvius, and so on.

There is a second nervous system, partly connected with the central nervous system and partly independent. This is the autonomic nervous system. It has nerve centres, called ganglia, located alongside the spinal cord. There are also ganglia in the head, the stomach, and other places. A blow in the region of the stomach ganglia knocks the wind out of you and you are breathless. The autonomic nervous system controls the working of the glands, the heart (the beating of the heart depends on a ganglion located there), and it is also closely connected with the feelings, as manifested in blushing, crying, etc. Some Yogis develop self-mastery to such a degree that they can influence the working of the autonomic nervous system.

Living depends on a constant reaction and adjustment to our environment. Without the complex nervous system this would be impossible. The ancient Yogis, in devising their disciplines, gave primary consideration to the maintenance of a healthy and efficient nervous system.

Hatha Yoga promotes the harmonious health of the internal organs and glands, the principal endocrine glands all being acted upon by the various postures.

Of these glands, George A. Dorsey, in his book *Why We Behave Like Human Beings*, says: "The secretions of the ductless glands are discharged direct into the blood, hence they are also called glands of internal secretion or endocrines (endon, within; krino, I separate). Endocrine secretions are chemical in nature and are usually called hormones (exciters). They are also called autacoid substances: from acos, a remedy—they act like drugs. They are, in fact drugs, some of them of astounding potency. In fact, no man-made drugs are so powerful as some we make in our own drug-store glands."

Rejuvenation

The work of the endocrine glands has a direct bearing on vitality and longevity. Hatha Yoga is the system par excellence of rejuvenation. Daily Yoga exercise not only wards off stiffness of the muscles and joints, one of the troubles of old age, but it also slows down the whole physiological ageing process. Biological and chronological time are two different things, the former varying with each individual. We age at different speeds. One man is a spent force at sixty, while another is comparatively fresh.

In *Man the Unknown*, Alexis Carrel writes:

"Inward time cannot be properly measured in units of solar time. However, it is generally expressed in days and years because these units are convenient and applicable to the classification of terrestrial events. But such a procedure gives no information about the rhythm of the inner processes constituting our intrinsic time. Obviously, chronological age does not correspond to physiological age. Puberty occurs at different epochs in different individuals. It is the same with menopause. True age is an organic and functional state. It has to be measured by the rhythm of the changes of this state. Such rhythm varies according to individuals. Some remain young for many years. On the contrary, the organs of others wear out early in life. The value of physical time in a Norwegian, whose life is long, is far from being identical with that in an Eskimo, whose life is short. To estimate true, or physiological, age, we must discover, either in the tissues or in the humours, a measurable phenomenon, which progresses without interruption during the whole life-time."

Of equal importance with the benefits to bodily health and efficiency that come from Hatha Yoga practice is the calming and integrating influence on the personality. For Hatha Yoga is a system of bodily purification, leading naturally to Raja Yoga, which is a technique of self-development and conscious evolution.

Tranquillity of mind is of as much importance as bodily care if you wish to live a long and active life. Looking over some cuttings from my files under the heading "Longevity", I notice a frequently occurring answer to the reporter's inevitable question to the centenarian: "To what do you attribute your long life?" The most frequently given reply is "freedom from worry" . . . in other words, peace of mind.

Worry is a great killer. Dr. Kenneth Walker has written that it kills more people than cancer. So, too, does boredom. Old people should have as many interests as possible. Retirement should be taken as an opportunity, not for idleness, but for creative leisure.

Great ages are reached in the Yoga ashrams of the East, where lives of self-mastery and tranquillity are lived. Exact figures are difficult to obtain, but claims of up to two hundred years are made. In China, where meditation is an ancient art, the Taoists lived such long lives that the Emperor Ch-Hoang-Ti (221-209 B.C.) thought they must have a secret elixir and sent for it.

The influence of the emotions on health is now well-known to medical science. Emotional stress or conflict can cause not only minor ailments, but serious diseases. Hatha Yoga purifies the body. Raja Yoga purifies the mind and achieves emotional mastery. The renowned Hungarian neuropathist, Dr. Francis Volgyesi, once said: "Yoga is actually the primitive ancestor, thousands of years old, of the brand-new science that we call psycho-therapy."

To achieve that harmony with nature that is perfect health, the Hatha Yoga in India goes through a rigorous programme. He devotes his life to it, performing many of the exercises for hours daily. This arduous practice gives him a control over body and mind that is extraordinary. (For a fascinating account of what it is like to undergo full training under a guru (Yoga master) see Theos Bernard's works *Hatha Yoga* and *Heaven Lies Within Us.*)

It is doubtful whether there would be many readers willing to undertake such a programme even if they had the time to spare. However, in a later chapter will be shown how fifteen to thirty minutes daily can be utilized for a Yoga programme of immense benefit to bodily and mental health.

In Chapter IV are given the best known of the Yoga exercises. Scientific tests have been made with regard

II

YOGA HYGIENE AND DIET

The Six Purification Practices

The ancient Yogis were thorough in the matter of personal hygiene and they developed certain practices to rid the body of impurities. These show an understanding and control of the human body unknown in the West.

The six main purification practices of Yoga are: DHAUTI, BASTI, NETI, TRATAKA, NAULI and KAPALABHATI.

Nevertheless, be warned. Though described here as likely to be of interest, it must be pointed out that Dhauti, Basti, Neti and Trataka could be dangerous to bodily health unless practised under a Yoga expert.

In DHAUTI a long strip of cloth—surgical gauze three to four inches in width will do—is swallowed and allowed to rest in the stomach for some time before pulling it out. The cloth may be soaked in warm water or milk before being 'eaten' bit by bit. Swallowing only two or three feet at first, it is possible when the lining of the throat becomes accustomed to the practice to take in fifteen feet or more. At first there is a desire to vomit but this passes. Several weeks of practice may be necessary before success is achieved. The cloth is allowed to remain in the stomach for ten to fifteen minutes before being pulled out. If it remains longer than twenty minutes it will commence to pass through the body.

Dhauti removes phlegm, bile and other impurities from the stomach and is said to cure many diseases. The *Hatha Yoga Pradipika*, one of the best known Yoga source books, says: "there is no doubt that cough, asthma, enlargement of the spleen, leprosy, and twenty kinds of diseases born of phlegm disappear by the practice of Dhauti Karma."

An alternative with similar benefits is to drink several glasses of warm water and salt until you vomit and empty the stomach (vamana dhauti).

By controlling the sphincters of the anus and performing nauli which creates a vacuum in the rectum water can be taken into the colon. The ancient Yogis performed this practice squatting in lakes or pools of water. The *Hatha Yoga Pradipika* recommends the use of a pipe, six inches long, half an inch wide, half inserted into the anus, while squatting in navel-deep water. But adepts may dispense with any aids whatever, relying on a powerful muscular control of the isolated abdominal recti muscles (nauli, to be described later) and the anal sphincters. The two recti-muscles are alternately relaxed and contracted in a churning action that assists thorough washing of the colon.

Modern colon irrigators make the practice of BASTI

unnecessary,* but it does show the extent to which the Yogi understands his body and has control over it.

NETI is a practice for cleaning the head sinuses. A piece of soft cord or warm water may be used. If the former, the cord is passed through one nostril and out of the mouth. The cord is slowly drawn back and forth for a time, then repeated through the other nostril. An alternative is to sniff water through the nostrils and expel it from the mouth (vyut-krama). It is possible to reverse this process and take the water through the mouth and expel it from the nostrils (sit-krama). An unpleasant sensation is experienced at first but passes away if the cleansing exercise is persisted in.

The *Gheranda Samhita* claims that "by this practice of Yoga one becomes like the god Cupid. Old age never comes to him and decrepitude never disfigures him. The body becomes healthy, elastic, and disorders due to phlegm are destroyed."

TRATAKA consists of staring without blinking at a candle flame or other mildly bright object. The Yogi continues until the eyes tire and begin to water, then ends the exercise and washes the eyes with cold water. The source books claim that this practice strengthens the eyes, can induce clairvoyance, and "should be kept secret very carefully, like a box of jewellery."

In my 'teens I was a member of a body-building gymnasium and as well as developing my muscles

---

* The natural Yoga method, however, is said to result in a more complete cleansing.

I learnt something of the technique of muscle control. One of the more sensational controls was to retract the muscles of the abdominal area and then isolate the two recti muscles. I practised every morning and evening in front of a bedroom mirror until I had mastered the control. To me at the time it was just a trick. A year or two later I discovered that what I was doing was the centuries old Yoga practice of NAULI.

Nauli cannot be performed until the first stage, UDDIYANA, has been perfected. Though it is described here, Uddiyana can be counted as one of the physical exercises (Asanas). Stand with feet apart and knees slightly bent. Lean forward, arching the back a little, and place your hands on your thighs just above the knees. Exhale all possible air from the lungs (it is important that this exhalation should be complete). Now pull your abdominal muscles upwards and backwards towards the spine. Concentrate on your solar-plexus and pull it as far into your thoracic cavity as possible. Hold for a couple of seconds then relax the muscles and let them return to their original position. Perform several times on one exhalation. As the muscles become stronger and more accustomed to the exercise you should be able to perform ten to twenty repetitions to one exhalation. This is called a round and a rest can be taken before another round. One to three rounds will be enough for most readers, but the

Indian Yogi thinks nothing of doing a thousand or
more repetitions.

Once Uddiyana has been mastered
NAULI can then be attempted. Having
exhaled and performed a full re-
traction, use pressure from your hands
on your thighs to assist in isolating the
two central recti abdominal muscles
which will sit out in a thin wedge.
Later you may be able to isolate each
of the recti muscles separately. By
alternately relaxing and contracting
the right and left recti the abdominal
muscles can be made to roll from side
to side in a wave-like motion.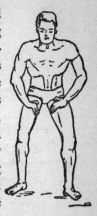

These controls are well worth mastering. Do not
worry if the second stage does not come easily to you.
Concentrate on performing uddiyana correctly and
the control of the recti will come later. Take it easy
at first and avoid strain. Practise before a mirror.

We have already seen the hygienic purpose behind
nauli, but uddiyana and nauli are highly valuable
exercises in themselves, being the finest known for
promoting and maintaining the health and vigour of
the abdominal region. Those who practice them are
unlikely to suffer from constipation, indigestion,
obesity, and diseases of the stomach.

KAPALABHATI is a breathing exercise for purifying
the nerve channels (nadis) and will be described in a
later chapter.

Oral Hygiene

As well as performing the six cleansing exercises the Yogi gives attention to the cleanliness of his mouth. He rinses his mouth with water and cleans the root of his tongue and his gums by massaging them with the tips of the first and second fingers of one hand. The teeth should be kept clean and periodically examined by a dentist.

Diet

It should be obvious that if you are not to jeopardize the vitality that Yoga promotes you must give attention to how and what you eat.

Here, moderation is the rule. The Yogi is advised at a main meal to fill half his stomach with food, one quarter with water, and keep one quarter empty. What this means is that at any meal you should eat enough to satisfy your hunger, but not so much as to give a gorged feeling.

Recommended Foods

The *Hatha Yoga Pradipika* lists the following foods as being "very beneficial to those who practise Yoga": wheat, rice, barley, good corns, milk, ghee, sugar, butter, sugar candy, honey, dried ginger, tonics, some vegetables, pure water.

And the *Gheranda Samhita* advises: rice, barley or wheaten bread, Mudga and Masa beans, jack-fruit, the jujube, the bonduc nut, cucumber, plantain, fig, green, fresh vegetables, black vegetables, patola leaves.

Injurious Foods

The *Hatha Yoga Pradipika* says that the following foods are harmful to a Yogi: rape seed, intoxicating liquors, oil cake, garlic, onion, plums, fish, meat, curds. It also advises against foods too bitter, salty, hot, fermented, or which have had to be heated again.

The *Gheranda Samhita* prohibits, at least in the beginning of Yoga practice, all bitter, acid, salt, pungent and roasted things, curd, whey, heavy vegetables, wine, palm nuts, over-ripe jack-fruit, pumpkins, gourds, berries and onions.

Some Simple Rules

The above advice from the Sanskrit texts is given as a matter of interest, but was of course meant for the Indian Yogi living a life of austerity and self-discipline. The following simple dietary rules are recommended to Western readers who wish to achieve sound health and obtain the best results from their Yoga practice.

(a). Keep your diet as natural as possible. To titillate the palate many of our foods are refined and chemically treated to a point where valuable nutrients are lost. Eat plenty of green vegetables and fresh fruit, cutting down on the starchy carbohydrates which overburden the Western diet. Vegetables and fruit keep bloodstream and skin healthy. Vitamin A, which improves vision and resistance to disease, is found in green vegetables, the best sources being watercress, spinach, cabbage and peas. Fresh fruits are the best sources of vitamin C, which keeps gums and teeth healthy, aids the healing of wounds, and protects us from the disease scurvy. Green vegetables also are rich in vitamin C.

(b). Eat brown wholemeal bread in preference to white. The beneficial nutrients of wheat are mostly lost in the process of refining.

(c). Drink plenty of milk. It is a rich source of calcium, phosphorus, potassium, sodium, and vitamins A and D. Vitamin D maintains the health of the bones and teeth, and protects us from rickets and osteomalacia.

(d). Eat plenty of cheese. It supplies body-building protein to the diet, and is a rich source of vitamin A, B2 (Riboflavin), niacin (nicotinic acid) and vitamin D. Vitamin B2 supplies energy and keeps complexion, eyes and nerve-tissues healthy. It is also found in yeast, milk, yoghourt, eggs and brown bread. Niacin is needed for efficient working of the heart, nerves, muscles and digestive system. It also protects us from pellagra.

(e). Masticate your food thoroughly. Yogis attach great importance to this—indeed they consider how to eat to be of almost as much importance as what to eat. Solid foods should be broken down and reduced to a liquid before passing into the stomach. This initial breaking down takes place in the mouth through chewing and the action of the saliva. Mastication is a necessary part of the digestive processes and should not be hurried or neglected.

(f). Do not eat when excited or emotionally upset. Emotional excitement impedes the flow of gastric juices in the stomach, resulting in indigestion. Other causes are lack of exercise, overeating, anxiety, and too much of the wrong foods—spices, pastries and fries. People with sedentary occupations are prone to stomach troubles. They should get as much fresh air and exercise as possible in their leisure time.

(g). Include some roughage in your diet. This prevents constipation. Foods containing a high percentage of roughage are brown bread, fresh and dried fruits, onions, cabbage, lettuce, spinach and cereals. Lack of exercise causes constipation—you will have little trouble in this respect if you regularly perform the Yoga Asanas.

(h). Do not overeat. Give your digestive processes a chance to do their work. Leave a quarter of your stomach free. A meal should be of sufficient bulk to satisfy hunger, but not to over-tax the digestive and eliminative organs. If you masticate properly you will obtain more nourishment from less food than you are used to now. Overeating is the principal cause of obesity. The overweight are prone to many complaints and diseases, diseases of the liver, kidneys and heart, diabetes, gout, high blood-pressure, digestive disorders. If you are overweight, cut down drastically on the carbohydrate foods: bread, pastry, flour, cakes, sweets, potatoes, etc. In their place substitute cheese, eggs, fruit, vegetables, nuts and yoghourt. The Yoga Asanas and breathing exercises are excellent for normalizing the figure.

(i). Drink plenty of water and fruit juices between meals.

III

YOGA POSTURES (ASANAS)

Yogic physical exercises—actually they are postures to be held for a certain length of time without repetitions—are unrivalled as a means of improving bodily health and suppleness. Their superiority over other systems—callisthenics, weight-lifting, gymnastics, etc. —lies in the fact that they aim at promoting the health and efficiency of the vital internal organs. In devising these postures the ancient Yogis displayed once again their profound knowledge of the human body. In particular, they bore in mind the need for keeping the spine, nerves and glands in healthy condition, thus giving organic vigour to the whole body.

Use commonsense when first attempting these postures. If you doubt the suitability of any of them consult your doctor. A person with high blood-pressure or heart ailment should leave out the Head Stand. Women should not do Yoga exercise during pregnancy or the menstrual periods. If, however, you are of normal health and suppleness you can attempt all the asanas right away, provided you are careful not to over-strain your body. Be content to progress gradually.

There are a number of Yoga postures which are

extremely contorting; these are given under the heading of "Advanced Postures". Correct performance of even the simplest poses will not be easy at first, however, especially if you have not led an athletic life or are carrying considerable surplus fat. Remember that the attempt is doing you good; and if you are inclined to be obese Yoga will soon normalize your figure.

Perform several of these postures daily. You will soon come to like them and will not wish to miss your daily session.

The Shoulder Stand Posture (Sarvangasana)

Most readers will be familiar with the 'bicycle' exercise, a favourite of athletes and sportsmen, in which you lie on your back and, supporting your hips with your hands, perform a pedalling action with your feet. The Shoulder Stand Posture is somewhat similar, but the legs are kept straight and the pose held.

Lie on your back on the floor. A rug or folded

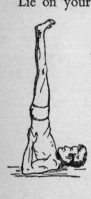

blanket can be used for comfort. The arms are kept alongside the body with the palms of the hands flat on the ground.

Keeping your legs together, raise them slowly until they are at right angles to the floor. The movement is continued by raising legs, hips and trunk into a vertical position. Place your hands on your hips and support the posture with the upper arms and elbows. Legs and back should be vertical and only the head, upper back and upper arms and elbows should be touching the ground. The upper chest will press against your chin. In this position try as if to touch the ceiling with your toes.

The position should be held for as long as you can do it comfortably, working up to several minutes with practice. Those of my readers who are athletic may like to dispense with the arm support after a while.

BENEFITS

Sarvangasana has a beneficial effect on the endocrine glands, especially the thyroid.

It tones up the whole nervous system.

It stretches the muscles of the legs, back, abdomen and neck.

It stretches the spine.

It improves circulation and sends a rich flow of blood to the spine and brain.

It reduces excess fat.

It is a wonderful rejuvenator.

The Plough Posture (Halasana)

If in the Shoulder Stand Pose you swing over your feet and legs until your toes touch the ground behind your head you will be in the Plough Posture, one of the finest of the Yoga asanas. It received its name because of a resemblance to the shape of an Indian plough.

Keep your arms stiff with the palms of your hands pressed against the ground. Your legs should be together and locked at the knees. When your toes touch the ground, attempt to push them as far as possible towards the wall behind your head.

You will not find this posture easy to attain, but keep trying. At first you will only be able to hold the position for a few seconds, but eventually you should manage thirty seconds or more.

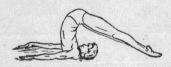

BENEFITS

Halasana promotes suppleness of the spine and helps maintain its natural curve.

It tones up the nervous system.

It stretches and makes more supple almost all the body muscles.

It exercises the abdomen and prevents disorders of the stomach.

It improves the circulation and sends a rich flow of blood to the spine.

It is one of the best movements for normalizing the obese figure and it rejuvenates the whole body.

The Inverted Body Posture (Sirsasana)

This is the Yoga "Head Stand".

If you wish, you can perform this pose against a wall or locked door, using a soft cushion to protect

your head. The adept will spurn
such aids, but it is a great help to the
beginner to have the fear of over-
balancing removed. Part of the pressure on the head can be shared by the
hands.

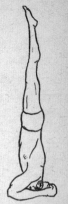

Thirty seconds should be long enough
to hold the pose at first, until the body
gets used to the inverted position. Each
day you can add one or two seconds.
until you can comfortably perform for
several minutes. Progress gradually, ending the posture if you begin to feel too much strain.
You will probably feel a slight giddiness on returning
to the perpendicular, but this quickly passes. A simple
and non-strenuous way of receiving most of the
benefits of Sirsasana is to use a Slant Board. Relax for
a few minutes on a board slanted so as to have your
feet higher than your head.

BENEFITS

Sirsasana sends a rich flow of refreshing blood to the
brain.

It relaxes body and mind.

It improves concentration.

It keeps you youthful. Yogis claim that it banishes
wrinkles and grey hair.

It normalizes your weight.

It improves body metabolism

The Bow Posture (Dhanurasana)

Lie flat on your stomach. Stretch your arms back and, raising your heels, grasp both ankles. Pulling with your arms, lift the legs as high as possible at the same time arching the front part of the body. It is as if you were trying to touch the back of your head with the soles of your feet.

This pose is difficult and at first you will probably have to keep your legs a little apart. Later you should be able to keep your legs together throughout.

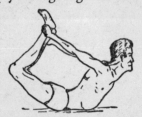

BENEFITS

Dhanurasana stretches and makes the spine more supple.

It tones up the nervous system.

It stretches the muscles of the abdomen, back, legs, arms and neck.

It improves the efficiency of the liver, kidneys and glands.

It improves the digestion.

It is one of the finest correctives for bad posture.

The Cobra Posture (Bhujangasana)

Lie face downwards, the palms of the hands resting on the ground level with the shoulders. Your forehead should also be touching the ground and your legs are kept stiff and together throughout the movement.

Slowly raise your head upwards and backwards. Face, neck and trunk will follow gradually. In the final position, which should be held, your arms will be straight and your head thrown back so that the eyes look at an angle towards the ceiling. In this pose the reason for the name 'Cobra' is obvious.

The important thing in performing the exercise is to put as much work as possible on to the spine. Of course you will find that you have to use your arms to assist. Indeed at first they will be doing most of the work. With practice it is possible for some people to dispense altogether with the aid of the arms.

Remember that the movement should be a slow, smooth one. There must be no jerking or straining.

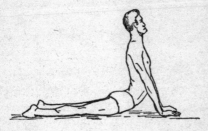

BENEFITS

Bhujangasana strengthens and promotes the health and suppleness of the spine.

It improves the efficiency of the nervous system.

It stretches the muscles of the abdomen, back, arms and neck.

It improves body metabolism.
It corrects bad posture.

The Posterior Stretch Posture
(Paschimatanasana)

This is similar to the well-known 'sit-up' exercise. You will find that a large number of the exercises popular with physical-culturists in the West are taken from Yoga. Paschimatanasana differs from an ordinary sit-up in that the movement is continued until the face comes close to the knees and this position is then held. Many Yogis acquire such suppleness that they can actually rest their faces on their knees.

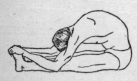 Lie flat on your back, legs outstretched and together. Sit up slowly and smoothly keeping the legs steady. Only the upper body moves. Exhale and carry the movement on in an effort to touch your knees with your face. At the same time stretch your arms forward and catch your toes (or your ankles if you are not very supple). Hold the position for several seconds, adding seconds as the position becomes more comfortable.

BENEFITS

Paschimatanasana works the spine in an opposite direction from that of bhujangasana and has similar results in promoting its health, strength and suppleness.

It stretches the muscles of the back, abdomen, arms and legs.

It aids digestion.

It removes surplus fat.

It is claimed in a Yoga source book that this asana "kindles gastric fire, reduces obesity and cures all diseases of men."

Standing Posterior Stretch (Padhahasthasana)

This is, as its name indicates, the posterior stretch performed in a standing position. The 'toes touch' we were taught as children has been taken from this asana. It differs in that you do not perform repetitions, but hold the pose for as many seconds as is comfortable. Again the face can be brought right down to the knees.

BENEFITS

As for Paschimatanasana.

ADVANCED POSTURES

The Locust Posture (Salabhasana)

Lie full length, face downwards on floor. The arms

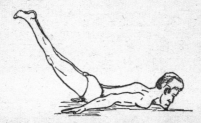

rest alongside the body with the knuckles down. The soles of the feet are upturned. Pressing with the arms and using the lower back muscles, raise the legs towards the ceiling. Hold for a few seconds. This is a vigorous exercise, benefiting the abdomen and lower back. The action resembles that of the locust.

The Peacock Posture (Mayurasana)

This is another vigorous exercise that will appeal to gymnasts. Commence from a kneeling position with knees spread apart. Place palms of hands together on the floor with fingers pointing towards your feet. The wrists should be touching. Lean forward on the hands with the elbows resting against the stomach. Now bring body weight forward and straighten legs until the body balances in a straight line on the hands and elbows. Hold for a few seconds. The abdominal area greatly benefits and is strengthened by this

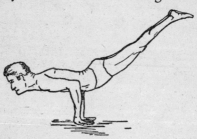

exercise. The *Hatha Yoga Pradipika* says of it : "This asana soon destroys all diseases and removes abdominal disorders, and also those arising from irregularities of phlegm, bile and wind, digests unwholesome food taken in excess, increases appetite and destroys the most deadly poison."

The Twist Posture (Ardha-Matsyendrasana)

Sit on the floor with your legs outstretched. Bend the left leg and place its heel into the crutch as in the first stage of Siddhasana. But this time the right foot is brought right across the left leg and placed on the floor outside it. The left hand grasps the toes of the right foot from outside the right knee. Trunk and head are twisted right round to do this, and the free right arm is bent across the lower back with palm outwards. This works the spine from a new angle, since it is twisted laterally.

Hold the pose for a few seconds at first, increasing to one to two minutes. Perform the twist to the other side to complete the exercise.

Patience and perseverence bring success in this posture but those who find it impossible can achieve a similar effect by sitting on a chair, twisting round and grasping the ends of the chair back with both hands. Keep legs and hips steady. Twist head and trunk right round as far as they will comfortably go.

Ardha-Matsyendrasana has a beneficial effect on the nervous system and on stomach, kidneys, liver, etc.

The Adamant Posture (Vajrasana)

Kneel with knees together and buttocks resting on your feet, the soles of which are turned uppermost. Rest the palms of your hands on their corresponding knees. The head is held erect and the back straight. This should not present any great difficulty, but this pose is the starting position for the advanced exercise of supta-vajrasana.

The Pelvic Posture (Supta-Vajrasana)

From the vajrasana posture slowly bend backwards, keeping the legs steady. Arms and elbows will have to be employed as an aid for most people. Lower the shoulders until they rest firmly on the floor. The arms may then be stretched full length beyond the head, palms up.

Hold for thirty seconds adding fifteen seconds each week until you can rest comfortably in this posture for two minutes.

Supta-Vajrasana has a beneficial stretching action on thighs and stomach. It prevents constipation and aids digestion. It enlarges the rib-box, and removes surplus fat.

The Fish Posture (Matsyasana)

First take up the Lotus Posture (page 73) then lean back until the body is supported by the top of the head and grasp your feet with your hands. The back should be fully arched and chest thrown out. In this posture you can float easily on the sea. Physical-culturists will recognize its similarity to the 'Wrestler's Bridge'. The neck, brain, chest, spine and stomach all benefit.

The Adept Posture (Baddha Padmasana)

Sit in the Lotus Pose, cross arms behind your back and grasp toes. This means that you grasp your right foot with your right hand and your left foot with your left hand.

The Cock Posture (Kukkutasana)

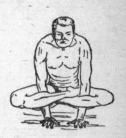

In Padmasana, your feet crossed on to your thighs, thrust your hands between knees and thighs and stand on your hands. This is a spectacular pose.

The Tortoise Posture (Uttanakurmakasana)

From Padmasana, thrust hands between thighs and calves as in The Cock Posture, but instead of standing on your hands this time you grasp your neck and sit balanced on your buttocks and lower back.

Symbol of Yoga (Yoga Mudra)

From the seated Padmasana position, lean forward and try to touch the floor in front of you with your forehead. The arms are placed behind the back with one hand grasping the opposite wrist.

This posture benefits the abdomen and internal organs, as well as preventing constipation, stomach disorders and obesity.

The Mountain Posture (Parbatasana)

Seated in one of the meditative postures, stretch both arms towards the ceiling and bring the palms and fingers of your hands together directly above your head as in the attitude of prayer. Now stretch your finger-tips towards the ceiling as far as they will comfortably go. This pose resembles a mountain (parbat). The posture may be accompanied by deep breathing. Inhale and exhale slowly and evenly 5-10 times.

The stretching action benefits the trunk and abdominal muscles, strengthens the spine, tones up the nervous system, improves digestion, removes constipation. The breathing action strengthens the lungs and purifies the bloodstream.

The Wheel Posture (Chakrasana)

Lie flat on your back on the floor. Bending your knees, draw your heels in against your buttocks. At the same time bend your arms at the elbows and place the palms of your hands on the floor on either side of your head, with the fingers pointing back towards the heels. To do this you will probably have to raise your buttocks a little. Distribute your body weight on the soles of your feet and palms of your hands. Now raise your trunk upwards until feet and hands take the full strain and the back is fully arched. "The Wheel" will not be unfamiliar to keen gymnasts. It is a very strenuous exercise and should only be attempted by advanced students.

Chakrasana has a beneficial effect on the whole spinal column, strengthens the nervous system, prevents and cures abdominal disorders, and reduces surplus fat.

The Triangle Posture (Trikonasana)

Stand upright with feet widely spaced. Extend both arms in a line with the shoulders. This is the starting position. Bend slowly to the right until you touch your right foot with your right hand. To do this you will have to bend your right knee a little. Only the right leg bends, the left stays outstretched to maintain balance. The outstretched left arm points upwards at an angle roughly parallel with the angle of the left leg. Return to the starting position, pause a few seconds, then perform the movement to the left. Perform several repetitions to each side.

The spine, nervous system and abdomen all benefit from Trikonasana. It also keeps the figure slim and shapely.

The Knee and Head Posture (Janusirasana)

This is a one-legged Paschimatana. Sit on the floor with your legs together and outstretched. Bending the left leg at the knee, bring the left heel into the crotch, as for Siddhasana. The right leg is kept fully stretched. Exhale, lean forward and grasp your right foot with both hands. Lower your head between your arms and attempt to touch your right knee with your head.

Hold for several seconds, then sit up again and perform the exercise with your left leg.

Janusirasana strengthens abdomen, spine and legs. It makes the spine more supple and benefits the spinal nerves. It normalizes the figure.

The Scorpion Posture (Vrischikasana)

A very advanced exercise indeed, similar to the gymnastic 'Tiger Bend'. With forearms resting shoulder width on the floor, the Yogi raises his body and legs into an inverted position, then slowly lowers his feet until they rest on the top of his head. It would be dangerous for beginners or the unathletic to attempt this pose.

Vrischikasana benefits the whole body, strengthens the spinal nerves, makes the spine more supple, and removes surplus fat.

8,400,000 Asanas

In the *Gheranda Samhita* we read that "there are eighty-four hundreds of thousands of Asanas described by Siva. The postures are as many in number as there are living creatures in this universe."

The best of these, and those most suitable to the Occident, have been described in this chapter. Their practice will rejuvenate the body, reduce obesity, strengthen the muscles, make the spine and body more supple and elastic, tone up the nervous system, keep diseases at bay, prevent constipation and dyspepsia, keep the skin glowing and healthy and promote mental alertness and serenity.

Therapeutic Powers of the Asanas

Definite therapeutic powers are claimed for the Asanas, and the work of such institutions as the Yoga Research Laboratory at Lonavla, under the directorship of Srimat Kuvalayananda, has done much to put these claims on a scientific basis. The following are a list of common disorders and the Asanas best used for their relief or cure as given by Yoga experts.

ASTHMA : Matsyasana, Parbatasana, Salabhasana, Sarvangasana, Savasana.

BRONCHITIS: Matsyasana, Parbatasana, Salabhasana.

CONSTIPATION: Ardha-matsyendrasana, Halasana, Janusirasana, Matsyasana, Nauli, Padhahastasana, Paschimatanasana, Savasana, Trikonasana, Uddiyani, Yoga Mudra.

DIABETES: Ardha-Matsyendrasana, Halasana, Matsyasana, Mayurasana, Parbatasana, Paschimatanasana, Sarvangasana, Savasana, Yoga Mudra.

INDIGESTION: Ardha-Matsyendrasana, Bhujangasana, Halasana, Mayurasana, Nauli, Parbatasana, Paschimatanasana, Sarvangasana, Salabhasana, Savasana, Uddiyani, Yoga Mudra.

INSOMNIA: Bhujangasana, Halasana, Parbatasana, Paschimatanasana, Sarvangasana, Salabhasana, Savasana.

LUMBAGO: Halasana, Salabhasana, Savasana.

MENSTRUAL DISORDERS: Bhujangasana, Halasana, Matsyasana, Nauli, Padhahastasana, Paschimatanasana, Sarvangasana, Uddiyani.

NEURASTHENIA: Parbatasana, Paschimatanasana, Sarvangasana, Sirsasana, Savasana.

OBESITY: Bhujangasana, Halasana, Paschimatanasana Padhahastasana, Salabhasana, Uddiyani.

PILES: Halasana, Matsyasana, Sarvangasana.

RHEUMATISM: Ardha-Matsyendrasana, Janusirasana, Parbatasana, Paschimatanasana, Sarvangasana.

SCIATICA: Janusirasana, Padhahastasana, Paschimatanasana, Sarvangasana.

SEXUAL DEBILITY: Nauli, Sarvangasana, Uddiyani, Yoga Mudra.

VARICOSE VEINS: Sarvangasana, Sirsasana.

The Meditative Postures

There are four more Asanas which cannot be omitted from any work on Hatha Yoga. The first three are the meditative postures Sukhasana, Siddhasana and Padmasana. The Yogis attach great importance to these and they will be described in the chapter on Yoga Breathing (Pranayama).

The other Asana is Savasana (The Corpse Posture). The need for relaxation being so great in the West, a separate chapter will be given to this subject.

IV

YOGA RELAXATION (SAVASANA)

Western civilized man lives at a pace that would
have left his forefathers breathless and bewildered.
His nervous system is subjected to almost constant
strain. Under the stress of such a way of life it is not
surprising that his health is usually below par and that
diseases and complaints resulting from tension have
become so prevalent. It has been estimated by various
authorities that at least fifty per cent of the people who
visit doctors' consulting rooms suffer from neurasthenia rather than from any organic disorder.

One of the immediate benefits reported by people
taking up Yoga is that they feel more relaxed. This is
a natural result of sitting still in the asanas, of breath
control, thought control and meditation. Yoga
quickly calms the mind, relaxes the body.

The Corpse Posture

While all the eight limbs of Yoga have a relaxing
influence, the Yogi usually finishes his programme of
asanas with one especially designed to rest the body
and re-charge it with energy.

This is Savasana, or The Corpse Posture. It is of such
value in combating present-day stress and strain you

should perform it at any time you can during the day.

Lie flat on your back with legs outstretched. Close your eyes and remain completely still, as if dead. This means lying with your full weight. You must really 'let go'.

You cannot expect to attain complete relaxation at the first attempt. It is an art which has to be mastered and this may take weeks, even months. But all the time you will be benefiting.

At first you will find that an obstinate tension remains and the body muscles refuse to relax. You must mentally go over them from head to toe seeking tension and removing it wherever it is found. Follow a definite order in relaxing the various muscles and muscle groups. This order is given below.

(1). Scalp and forehead.
(2). Eyes and eyeballs.
(3). Jaw and mouth.
(4). Throat.
(5). Deltoids (Shoulders).
(6). Pectorals (Breasts).
(7). Biceps.
(8). Abdominals.
(9). Forearms.
(10). Hands and fingers.
(11). Extensors of the thighs (Front part of thighs).
(12). Feet and toes.
(13). Neck.

(14). Trapezius (On top of back, below the neck.)

(15). Latissimus dorsi (The two large wedge-shaped muscles covering the shoulder-blades).

(16). Triceps (Rear part of upper arms).

(17). Buttocks.

(18). Biceps of thighs (Rear parts of thighs).

(19). Calves.

You will note that even the eyes, fingers and toes are included. Every particle of tension must be removed from the body.

Ability to relax comes quickly if you can 'get the feel' of all nineteen muscles or muscle groups by alternately tensing and relaxing them. In this way you can talk to your muscles. Special muscle-control exercises for achieving this are given in the author's *The Art of Relaxed Living* (Thorsons Publishers Ltd.).

For this posture it is best to lie on the floor on a folded blanket. Collars, ties and other constricting clothing should be removed. You cannot relax if you feel uncomfortable in any way.

As you become more adept you will find that you will be able to relax with a fair degree of success even in a sitting position, something which you can utilize in travelling by bus or train to and from your place of employment.

There is no more efficacious way of combating tension than to have a daily relaxation period or periods. So from now on make it a rule to perform The Corpse Posture (Savasana) at least once every day.

V

YOGA BREATHING (PRANAYAMA)

Pranayama—from prana (the life breath) and ayama (pause)—is the Yoga science of breath control.

The ancient Yogis studied anatomy and explored body and consciousness to learn their secrets. One of the important things they discovered was the reciprocal relationship between the emotions and breathing. When we are excited our rate of respiration becomes faster. When we are composed, our breathing is slow, calm and rhythmical. The Yogi seeks by controlled, measured breathing to influence consciousness itself. By control of the breath the mind can be stilled and made one-pointed. Pranayama is a means to self-mastery and psychic powers.

Prana

It is necessary to point out that Prana, to the Yogi, means much more than mere breath. Prana is actually the power behind and within breath. The power of the atom is Prana. Thought is Prana. It is "the vital force in every being". It is cosmic energy. It pervades the whole universe. It is everywhere and through Pranayama we can tap this illimitable well of universal energy.

Vivekananda, in his *Raja Yoga*, says : "In this body of ours the breath motion is the 'silken thread'; by laying hold of and learning to control it we grasp the pack thread of the nerve currents, and from these the stout twine of our thoughts, and lastly the rope of Prana, controlling which we reach freedom.

"We do not know anything about our own bodies; we cannot know. At best we can take a dead body, and cut it in pieces, and there are some who can take a live animal and cut it in pieces in order to see what is inside the body. Still, that has nothing to do with our own bodies. We know very little about them. Why do we not? Because our attention is not discriminating enough to catch the very fine movements that are going on within. We can know of them only when the mind becomes more subtle and enters, as it were, deeper into the body. To get that subtle perception we have to begin with the grosser perceptions. We have to get hold of that which is setting the whole engine in motion; that is the Prana, the most obvious manifestation of which is the breath. Then along with the breath, we shall slowly enter the body, which will enable us to find out about the subtle forces, the nerve currents that are moving all over the body. As soon as we perceive and learn to feel them, we shall begin to get control over them, and over the body. The mind is also set in motion by these different nerve currents, so at last we shall reach the state of perfect control over the body and the mind, making both our servants. Knowledge is power; we have to get this power, so we must begin at the beginning, the Pranayama, restraining the Prana."

Breath is Life

To prepare the mind for the meditative exercises and disciplines, the Yogi seeks to control respiration, the body's key function and "the most obvious manifestation of Prana". Life is impossible without air. We can do without food and water for several days, but totally check our air supply and we are dead in a few minutes.

Our bodies need oxygen to burn up waste matter and purify the bloodstream. Civilized man has lost the art of breathing properly. His shallow breathing utilizes only about one-tenth of his lung capacity. The lack of oxygen from which he inevitably suffers is responsible for headaches, fatigue, lack of mental alertness. It is a contributory cause of that 'tired feeling' so many people complain of today. (A yawn is Nature's way of enabling us to get more oxygen when there is a lack of it.)

The Yoga breathing exercises, if performed sensibly and without strain, can be a means to greater bodily vitality, and can exert a beneficial influence over the emotions and the mind.

The Meditative Postures

For Pranayama and meditation the Yogis use certain seated postures which keep the body compact and perfectly steady. The three best known of these are Sukhasana, the Easy Posture; Siddhasana, the Perfect Posture; and Padmasana, the Lotus Posture.

The Perfect Posture (Sidhasana)

Bend the left leg and place the sole of the left foot against the perineum (between anus and scrotum). The right leg is brought across and the foot placed in the crevice between the calf and thigh of the left leg with the heel against the pubic bone.

The Lotus Posture (Padmasana)

Bending each leg at the knee, place each foot on the opposite thigh, soles upwards. This posture is that of the Yoga adept, and is obviously more difficult than Sidhasana.

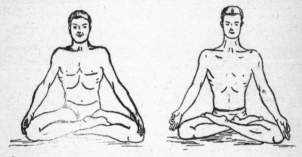

The Easy Posture (Sukhasana)

For most readers the Easy Posture will suffice. Sit on the floor with both legs stretched before you. Now bend one leg and place its foot under the thigh of the opposite leg. Then bend that leg and place it under the other leg.

These seated postures are practised by the Oriental from childhood and they are natural to him, but the Occidental often finds that his joints are too stiff to perform them at first. A lot will depend on age and suppleness. Do not use force. If the knees obstinately refuse to lower, leave it to time. Sitting on a thick book enables the position to be adopted more readily. The book can be dispensed with once proficiency has been attained. The knees should be wide-spaced and close to the ground. The head should be kept erect and the back straight. Once this is achieved a feeling of mastery and solidity is experienced. It is a relaxing and confident feeling that makes the trouble taken worth while.

If by any chance you cannot sit on the ground at all, use a stool or chair. The important thing is for the body to be perfectly steady, with the head, neck and back held in a straight line.

Note the position of the hands in the illustrations. The backs of the wrists rest on the knees and the first finger of each hand is bent and touches the thumb.

Before commencing Pranayama it is required that the body should be clean and free of impurities. Have a sponge down and clear the nostrils. Rinse your mouth with water and rub tongue and gums with your fingers.

At least two hours should have elapsed since a meal.

The exercises should be done in the open, before an open window, or at least in an airy room.

Wear loose fitting clothes, but don't risk catching cold. Remove constricting collars and ties.

The Cleansing Breath (Kapalabhati)

Kapalabhati does not really belong to Pranayama, but is one of the six purification practices (see Chapter II). It is designed to clear the sinuses and rid the nerve channels (nadis) of impurities and should precede the other breathing exercises.

As with all the breathing exercises given in this chapter it is best performed in one of the meditative postures.

Inhalation (puraka) and exhalation (rechaka) take place through the nose, the latter being accomplished by means of a quick and vigorous contraction of the abdominal muscles and diaphragm.

Take a deep breath through both nostrils, then pull in the abdominal muscles and diaphragm in a sharp instroke that forces the air out of your nose so fast as to be almost a sneeze. Immediately the exhalation is finished, inhale again.

Exhalation should take less time than inhalation. At the start do it ten times at the rate of two exhalations per second. This completes a round. Take a minute's rest, breathing normally, before commencing a further round.

You should be able to add to the size of a round

until you are doing twenty or more inhalations and exhalations. Speed too can be increased but this should never be at the expense of efficiency.

There is likely to be a slight soreness of the abdomen at first until the muscles strengthen. Daily practice of uddiyana as described in Chapter II will facilitate the performance of Kapalabhati.

BENEFITS:
Kapalabhati clears the nasal passages, cleanses the sinuses and nerve channels.

It enriches the bloodstream and improves circulation.

It rejuvenates and is said to prolong life.

It prepares the body for Pranayama.

Comfortable Pranayama (Sukh Purvak)

This is an easier and less strenuous cleansing exercise.

Sit in one of the meditative postures. Close the right nostril with your right thumb. Inhale slowly and evenly through the left nostril, filling the lower (often neglected) parts of the lungs, then the middle and upper lungs. There must be no forcing. Retain the air for a few seconds, closing the left nostril with the left thumb. This breath suspension the Yogi calls Kumbhaka. Then release the right nostril and exhale slowly through it.

Now repeat the process. Inhale through the right nostril, retain the air and exhale through the left nostril. This is one round.

The ratio favoured by the Yogis between puraka,

kumbhaka and rechaka is 1:4:2. That is to say, if you inhale for five seconds, you suspend the breath for twenty seconds, and exhale over a count of ten seconds. At first, however, it would be inadvisable to use such a ratio, gradually working up to it from ratios of 1:1:2 and 1:2:2. The breath must always be even and kept under perfect control.

BENEFITS:

Sukh Purvak aids digestion and improves the appetite.

It cleanses the nasal passages, and sinuses.

It tones up the nervous system.

It purifies and enriches the bloodstream.

It has a calming and concentrating effect on the mind.

The Bellows Breath (Bhastrika)

This breathing exercise is so named because it imitates the action of a blacksmith's bellows.

In Bhastrika you inhale and exhale at the rate of about one inhalation and exhalation per second. As in Kapalabhati the inhalation should be twice as long as the exhalation, which is assisted by a quick instroke of the abdominal muscles and diaphragm. It differs from Kapalabhati in that a suspension of breath (kumbhaka) is added at the end of each round. It also differs in a variation using alternate instead of both nostrils.

Ten exhalations will be enough for one round at first but later you should be able to manage comfortably sixty exhalations in a round of one minute. At the completion of each round perform a kumbhaka as follows—

Inhale deeply and slowly through the right nostril (pingala) until the lungs are comfortably filled. Retain the breath for some seconds, then exhale slowly through the left nostril (ida). When all the air has been expelled inhale through the same nostril. Suspend again. Exhale through the right nostril. This is done at the end of each round. When using one nostril the other is held closed with a finger or thumb.

Yoga literature contains several slight variations of technique. Sometimes the kumbhaka is described with the use of both nostrils.

The chief variation is to use alternate instead of both nostrils in the 'bellows' part of Bhastrika. Close your left nostril. Exhale through the right nostril. Inhale through the same nostril and exhale sharply through the left nostril. This means releasing the left nostril and at the same time closing the right. Immediately you have expelled the air through the left nostril you inhale through it and exhale through the right nostril, and so on.

BENEFITS :

Bhastrika is greatly favoured by Yogis as it is said to awaken the energy (kundalini) previously dormant in the body.

It removes the phlegm and cleanses the nerve channels.

It purifies the bloodstream.

It aids digestion.

It prevents and cures disease.

It warms the body.

It tones up the nervous system.

The Audible Breath (Ujjayi)

In Ujjayi you breathe through both nostrils. It differs from the other pranayamas in that the glottis remains half-closed during puraka and rechaka. This partial closure of the glottis produces a soft but clearly audible sound during breathing. The steadiness of this sound should be noted to see if the breathing is as smooth, slow and controlled as it should be.

Between inhalation and exhalation there is a suspension of breath which is assisted by the chin-lock (jalandhara). The chin is lowered and rested firmly in the jugular notch. The Yogis say that through kumbhaka, Prana can be sent to all parts of the body, "from the nails of the toes to the tips of the hair." Some of them develop the practice of breath suspension to such a degree that they can be buried for days without coming to any harm.

We can marvel at, but need not try to emulate, such feats. Do not try to prolong kumbhaka unduly. Besides the possibility of a strain of lungs or heart, if you suspend the breath over-long exhalation will not be under full control. The air will be expelled violently or jerkily instead of in the smooth, even manner required.

Ujjayi can be performed standing, and even when walking, as well as in the meditative postures. People whose leisure time is limited should watch out for opportunities to perform this breathing exercise in the course of their daily activities.

BENEFITS :

Ujjayi clears the head and removes phlegm from the throat.

It cleanses the nerve channels and tones up the whole nervous system.

It cures and prevents diseases like asthma and consumption.

It aids digestion and banishes dyspepsia.

It purifies the bloodstream.

It prolongs life.

Sitkari

In this pranayama the teeth are kept together and the air is inhaled through the mouth with a hissing sound.

Suspend the breath, using the chin lock.

Exhale through the nostrils.

BENEFITS :

Sitkari purifies the bloodstream.

It prevents and cures diseases.

It aids digestion.

It appeases hunger and quenches thirst.

It cools the body.

Sitali

In Sitali the tongue is protruded beyond the lips and folded into a trough.

Inhalation, suspension and exhalation are performed as in Sitkari.

BENEFITS :
As in Sitkari.

These are the most important exercises of Pranayama. Readers will be able to select two or three for daily practice. If performed carefully and as instructed, there will be an immediate increase in bodily vitality, and a tranquillizing effect on the mind will be produced. But forcing or long breath suspensions must be avoided.

The *Hatha Yoga Pradipika* makes this clear. "Just as lions, elephants and tigers are controlled by and by, so the breath is controlled by slow degrees, otherwise it kills the practiser himself. When Pranayama, etc., are performed properly, they eradicate all diseases, but an improper practice generates diseases. Hiccup, asthma, cough, pain in the head, the ears, the eyes; these and other various kinds of diseases are generated by the disturbances of the breath. The air should be expelled with proper tact, and should be filled in skilfully, and should be kept confined properly. Thus it brings success. When the nadis (nerve channels) become free from impurities, and there appear the outward signs of success, such as lean body and glowing colour, then one should feel certain of success.

By removing the impurities of the nadis the air can be restrained, according to one's wish, and the appetite is increased, the divine sound is awakened, and the body becomes healthy."

VI

MAKING THE MOST OF THE EXERCISES

How Much Time Is Needed?

You will naturally be wondering how much time you need devote to Yoga exercises to obtain benefit. Any time given to it will not be wasted, but for satisfactory results at least fifteen minutes daily should be given to the exercises of Part I.

There is an argument I hear over and over again: "I would like to have more vitality, better stamina, a shapelier and more youthful appearance, a tranquil mind . . . but I just haven't the time."

I don't think there is a person living—no matter how full his daily activities—who could not find time (and lots of it) for some worthwhile task.

Try this experiment. For one whole day, from rising in the morning to retiring to bed in the evening, write down how you spent every minute. At the end of the day you will be amazed to find the number of minutes, probably hours, that have been wasted on nothing of importance. This is true even of those people who claim that they never have a minute to spare. If you utilize this time and add to it an extra half-hour a day through rising that much earlier in the morning, you will, believe it or not, be 'making' several weeks extra time per year. Work it out for yourself.

This book has been written in the knowledge that most of its readers will be busy people, but the mere fifteen minutes or so extra time required daily for your yoga practice can be easily 'made', as I have shown, and surely are worth spending to achieve physical and mental health hitherto inconceivable.

Time and Place

Your daily Yoga practice may take place at any time you like provided at least two hours have elapsed since having a meal. A regular time each day should be fixed. Usually the most suitable times are in the morning on rising or before retiring to bed in the evening. Of these two the former is probably the better time as it gives a good start to the day. Exercises may be performed in the morning and meditation in the evening.

Wash yourself all over with cold or luke-warm water, followed by a good towelling so that the skin is clean and glowing.

You may then wish to perform neti as described in the chapter on Yoga Hygiene. Sniff warm water to which a little salt has been added up one nostril and expel it from the mouth. Do this a few times with alternate nostrils.

Follow this by brushing the teeth and rinsing your mouth. Wet the first and second fingers of either hand

and massage your gums and tongue with them. Fill your mouth with water two or three times and spit it out.

Place a folded blanket or rug on the floor of an airy, but not cold or draughty room. You can, of course, exercise outdoors if the weather is suitable. Wear as little clothing as possible, and that loose-fitting.

A 15 Minute Programme

The postures and breathing exercises lend themselves to a certain order which gives best results.

Here is a Yoga programme which makes the most of the exercises and including rest pauses takes only fifteen minutes.

Commence with Uddiyana (and Nauli when you can do it). It gives an internal massage to the abdominal area. Exhale and perform one to twenty contractions according to your ability. Remember that to do this successfully all possible air must be expelled from the lungs. Take fifteen seconds' rest then do another round. Later you should be able to add a third round.

This will be sufficient for ordinary purposes, but the advanced Yogi may practise until he is performing at least 750 contractions. Theos Bernard, who undertook the full Yogi discipline, under an Indian guru, reported in his *Hatha Yoga* that he practised Uddiyana twice a day, in the morning and late afternoon. He commenced with several rounds of ten contractions to the exhalation. Soon he increased the number of contractions to twenty and was doing ten rounds. He added five extra rounds each week until he passed the minimum 750 contractions. Bernard increased the contractions to fifty on each exhalation and ended up doing one thousand contractions twice a day, taking thirty to forty minutes.

He then began Nauli, isolating and rolling from side to side the rectus abdominus. He developed this exercise until he was able to perform a total of 750 isolations, twenty-five to each exhalation.

It should be remembered that Bernard was devoting his whole time, morning till night, to Yoga practice. And he states : "It is not necessary to carry these exercises to such extremes in order to obtain physical benefits. They were assigned to me as a preparation for the advanced practice of Yoga, and I had to master them before I was permitted to take up the next step. During this initial period, when I was learning techniques, I noted a sharper appetite, better vision, and better physical tone. All the muscles of my body were in good condition, hard and solid. I enjoyed excellent health and was free from all minor ailments of sedentary life."

The Postures

Begin the postures with THE SHOULDER-STAND (SARVANGASANA). Do it slowly and stretch your toes towards the ceiling. Hold for up to one minute. Lower the legs slowly to the ground.

Rest for fifteen seconds.

Raise your legs again and this time carry them over your head until the toes touch the floor beyond your head. You may find the PLOUGH POSTURE (HALASANA) difficult at first. Possibly you will have to spread your legs and bend them at the knees. At any rate hold whatever posture you can manage for up to one minute.

Rest again for fifteen seconds.

Turn over and do the COBRA POSTURE (BHUJANGASANA). Going into the posture should be a slow, smooth rising of the front part of the body with no more assistance from the arms than is absolutely necessary.

As you perform this, and all the other Asanas, have a mental picture of the good they are doing you, stretching the muscles and vertebrae, improving the circulation, toning up the nervous system, promoting strength, health and vitality.

Take fifteen seconds' rest after the Cobra, then turn over again on to your back so as to perform THE POSTERIOR STRETCH POSTURE (PASCHIMATANASANA). Even if you cannot get your face on to your knees without bending your legs remember that you are benefiting from the exercise. Hold the position for up to one minute.

Fifteen seconds' rest.

THE BOW POSTURE (DHANURASANA) will pull your spine in another direction than did Paschimatasana. This is not an easy pose, but continued practice will bring increased success.

Follow with fifteen seconds' rest.

THE HEAD STAND (SIRSASANA) can be done against a wall or locked door. The position will be strange to you at first, but when you begin to feel its benefits you will start enjoying the posture. Use a soft cushion for your head. This pose brings a copious flow of blood to the head, thus nourishing the brain cells.

People with high blood-pressure or heart complaints should not do Sirsasana, and elderly people may prefer the mild variation of lying at an angle with the feet raised higher than the head. When Dad puts his stockinged feet on the mantelpiece, he may not know it but he is relaxing the Yoga way.

Do not attempt to hold the inverted position for long periods. As soon as any discomfort is felt *slowly* lower your feet to the ground. I have known students continue until having blackouts, which is of course foolish and dangerous.

It is interesting to note, however, that Theos Bernard was set a standard of three hours. He began with ten seconds for the first week, adding thirty seconds each week until doing fifteen minutes. After many months he was able to hold the inverted posture for the required three hours at a stretch. This seems incredible, and Bernard's reactions are of interest. What is it like to stand on one's head for three hours? He says that on immediately taking up the pose his respiratory rate speeded up, then slackened again. For a while he felt very relaxed, then came a tendency to restlessness, followed by a copious flow of perspiration from face and body. This, he was told, was a danger signal, and he had then to stop. Later he was able to overcome this tendency.

Bernard found by this time that his greatest problem was mental rather than physical. He did not know what to do with his mind. His teacher told him to fix his gaze on a spot level with his eyes and concentrate his mind on it. When he did this time passed rapidly. He was also permitted to do a few movements with his legs when in the inverted posture.

The Breathing Exercises

Now adopt a seated cross-legged position for commencing the breathing exercises.

Start with the Cleansing Breath (Kapalabhati). You should be able to manage one inhalation and exhalation per second. Work up to twenty or more repetitions. Take a short rest then do another round.

After fifteen seconds' rest during which you can breathe normally, commence the Bellows Breath (Bhastrika). This can be done using both nostrils or alternate nostrils. When preceding it with Kapalabhati I prefer the alternate nostrils variation. Work up to twenty or more repetitions followed by a Kumbhaka. Avoid strain during the breath retention. Take a few seconds' rest, then do another round.

Again the rest pause of fifteen seconds.

Finish your Pranayama with the Audible Breath (Ujjayi). Remember that smoothness and control are required throughout if the maximum benefits are to be received. Continue Ujjayi for about a minute.

In all the breathing exercises have a mental picture of your body being flooded with the life-force of Prana. Feel the Prana being carried on the enriched bloodstream to every cell in your body.

Ujjayi completed, you should finish the programme with Yoga Relaxation (Savasana). Even two or three minutes' high-quality relaxation can make a pleasant ending to the Yoga session and you should get up feeling ready to tackle whatever work and responsibilities the day has in store for you.

The programme just described will take only fifteen minutes, including the rest pauses between exercises.

If any day you have less time to spare a still beneficial schedule would be Shoulder Stand or Head Stand, Cobra or Bow, Posterior Stretch, Comfortable Pranayama or Cleansing Breath.

And if you have only five minutes to spare, perform the Cat Stretch and Comfortable Pranayama or the Cleansing Breath.

The Yoga Cat Stretch

This is one of the most complete exercises known to man, a combination of several asanas and a 'work-out' in itself. The ancient Yogis first devised it after studying the stretching actions of the jungle animals. You can observe the domestic cat performing similar movements.

Stand with feet together, then lean forward and place the palms of your hands on the floor at shoulder width. Arms and legs should be stiff; the buttocks are held as high as possible and the body supported on the toes and hands. Keep your chin tucked in against your chest so that you are gazing at your feet. This is the first position.

Bending your arms, bring your head forward and shoulders downwards in a sweeping, circular motion. The chest should sweep low and touch the floor as it passes between the hands. Straighten your arms. At the completion of the circular motion your back should be arched with your head pressing backwards, chin up and eyes staring at the ceiling. Use your locked arms to push the body upwards and backwards. You will recognize this position as being identical with the Cobra Posture. Hold for a few seconds before returning to the original position by reversing the movements described.

Perform several repetitions.

Regular Practice Essential

Try never to miss your daily Yoga practice. After a few days I am certain you will not want to miss it. Indeed you will probably want to give extra time to it. If you do so, you may like to split the postures and breathing into separate periods. Ten to fifteen minutes could be given to the postures in the morning and ten to fifteen minutes to Yoga breathing in the evening. A few minutes' Pranayama before retiring will not only help you get to sleep but improve its quality as well.

During the day you will probably find opportunities for doing a few minutes' Uddiyana, Savasana, Sirsasana or Ujjayi (remember that this can be done walking). Time spent in Yoga practice is never wasted.

FIFTEEN MINUTE YOGA EXERCISE PROGRAMME

	POSTURES	MINUTES
1.	Abdominal Contraction (Uddiyana)	1
2.	The Shoulder Stand (Sarvangasana)	1
3.	The Plough (Halasana)	1
4.	The Cobra (Bhujangasana)	1
5.	The Posterior Stretch (Paschimatanasana)	1
6.	The Bow (Dhanurasana)	1
7.	The Head Stand (Sirsasana)	1

BREATHING EXERCISES

8.	The Cleansing Breath (Kapalabhati)	1
9.	The Bellows Breath (Bhastrika)	1
10.	The Audible Breath (Ujjayi)	1
11.	The Corpse Posture (Savasana)	2
	Rest pauses between exercises	3
	Total time	15 min.

TEN MINUTE YOGA EXERCISE PROGRAMME

POSTURES	MINUTES
1. Abdominal Contraction (Uddiyana)	1
2. The Shoulder Stand (Sarvangasana) or The Head Stand (Sirsasana) ..	1
3. The Cobra (Bhujangasana) or The Bow (Dhanurasana) ..	1
4. The Posterior Stretch (Paschimatanasana)	1

BREATHING EXERCISES

5. The Cleansing Breath (Kapalabhati) or Comfortable Pranayama (Sukh Purvak)	2
6. The Corpse Posture (Savasana) ..	2½
Rest pause between exercises ..	1½

Total time   ..   .. 10 min.

FIVE MINUTE YOGA EXERCISE PROGRAMME

POSTURE	MINUTES
1. The Yoga Cat Stretch	2½

BREATHING EXERCISE

2. Comfortable Pranayama (Sukh Purvak) or The Cleansing Breath (Kapalabhati)	2½

Total time   ..   .. 5 min.

FIFTEEN MINUTE YOGA EXERCISE PROGRAMME FOR WOMEN

	POSTURES	MINUTES
1.	The Shoulder Stand (Sarvangasana)	1½
2.	The Cobra (Bhujangasana)	1½
3.	The Posterior Stretch (Paschimatan-asana)	1½
4.	The Bow (Dhanurasana)	1½
5.	The Mountain (Parbatasana)	1½

BREATHING EXERCISES

6.	The Cleansing Breath (Kapalabhati)	1½
7.	The Audible Breath (Ujjayi) ..	1½
8.	The Corpse Posture (Savasana) ..	2½
	Rest pauses between exercises ..	2
		—
	Total time	15 min.

PART TWO

SELF-REALIZATION THROUGH RAJA YOGA

With the sword of the understanding of thyself thou shalt rend asunder in thy heart every doubt arising from ignorance, and thou shalt achieve thy permanence in Yoga.

Bhagavad Gita

It (is) astonishing that Western reason has taken so little into account the experimental research of Indian Raja-yogins, and that it has not tried to use the methods of control and mastery, which they offer in broad daylight without any mystery, over the one infinitely fragile and constantly warped instrument that is our only means of discovering what exists.

Romain Rolland

VII

THE ROYAL PATH (RAJA YOGA)

Raja Yoga

Hatha Yoga brings the body into harmony with the universe. The postures, breathing exercises, etc., have a calming influence on the mind and prepare it for the disciplines of Raja Yoga—the Royal Path. Hatha Yoga is a preparation for the conquest of consciousness, the mind's turbulence being easiest curbed and its energies concentrated in a strong body.

Alain Danielou, in a work on the different Yoga ways, says: "The movements of the mind are the cause of man's bondage. The action of his intellect is the instrument of his freedom. That particular mode of action by which the intellect stills the movements of the mind is known as the Royal Way to reintegration. This is the highest form of Yoga, all other forms being preparatory."

Self-Mastery

If you are already carrying out daily Yoga practice you will have experienced its beneficial influence on the mind. The steady, natural postures and smooth, measured Pranayama have a calming and controlling effect on thought and emotion. The meditative exercises of Raja Yoga will complete this mastery.

It takes but a little self-observation to see just how limited is the control over our minds. Raja Yoga teaches mastery of one's mind and self by psychic exercises aimed at controlling and subduing the thought waves or vrittis. The word vritti means literally "a whirlpool"—and that is just what most people's minds are like.

Harmonious health is impossible if the emotions are not under control. Emotional stresses—worry, fear, frustration, insecurity—are now known to be responsible for such diverse complaints as peptic ulcer, coronary thrombosis, high blood-pressure, tuberculosis, pneumonia, appendicitis, diabetes, asthma, schizophrenia. It has been estimated that in America more than half the people seeking the services of doctors suffer from emotionally induced complaints.

When subjected to stress, the body's glands, in particular the adrenals, release chemicals into the bloodstream which act as resistance mobilizers. When the stress is prolonged, these chemicals turn traitor and can cause serious damage to vital organs. Also bodily resistance to other attacks is lowered.

We can experience for ourselves the harmful and unpleasant effects of such an emotion as anger—the eyes protrude, the face burns, blood pressure rises, the fists clench, the stomach muscles contract. Dark emotions like fear, anxiety, jealousy, and hatred poison the bloodstream and destroy health and peace of mind. Medical science now recognizes them as killers.

But the bright emotions making for harmony—love, joy, hope, etc.—have a beneficial influence on bodily health. The dark emotions contract; the bright emotions expand. Supreme among the latter is Love, which if supported by Courage will protect you from the stresses of civilization and lead to a richer and fuller life.

All Yoga practice has the effect of stilling the mind's turbulence and holding the flame of the passions steady. A considerable measure of Detachment (Vairagya in Yogic terminology) is built up. In Vairagya one does not react automatically to stimuli or impulses, but first relates them to an objective "I" who decides what the course of action should be. This means that you do not give way to temper or any of the destructive dark emotions. In fact the "I" kills them before the bodily reaction of flushed skin, tensed muscles and adrenalin-saturated blood has time to take place. Most people are slaves to environmental changes. Even the weather can affect them. The "I" of ten o'clock is not the "I" of eleven o'clock; it may not even be the "I" of one minute past ten, for environmental change of stimuli taking only a split second could trigger off a new mood, a different-coloured "I". Yoga puts you in touch with your objective "I", gives you a permanent centre of gravity. When things are examined objectively, without heat or passion, one ceases to become attached to them.

They lose their power to disturb or inflame. Normally it takes much time for old wounds to heal. Such is the miracle of Vairagya that they heal in a matter of seconds.

All this makes for inner tranquillity. The Yogi may continue to live an active civilized life, but he will do so calmly and steadily. Sri Aurobindo, in his *Basis of Yoga*, has this to say of the calm mind that results from self-training:

"In the calm mind, it is the substance of the mental being that is still, so still that nothing disturbs it. If thoughts or activities come, they do not arise at all out of the mind, but they come from outside and cross the mind as a flight of birds crosses the sky in a windless air. It passes, disturbs nothing, leaving no trace. Even if a thousand images, or the most violent events pass across it, the calm stillness remains as if the very texture of the mind were a substance of eternal and indestructible peace. A mind that has achieved this calmness can begin to act, even intensely and powerfully, but it will keep its fundamental stillness—originating nothing for itself, but receiving from Above and giving a mental form without adding anything of its own, calmly, dispassionately, though with the joy of the Truth and the happy power and light of its passage."

We live in exciting but dangerous times. If we are to come through unscathed we will need the self-mastery that comes from peace of the spirit and having a permanent centre of gravity. The average person does not know the inner peace and integration of the

Yogi. His thoughts are leaves driven hither and thither by the wind of his desires. Through Raja Yoga faithfully practised the mind can be stilled, thoughts controlled, selected and directed at will. The value of such a mastery in civilized life is obvious.

La Rue puts it: "Health is wealth; but the very exuberance of bodily health may be a curse without proper mental control. All health that is not ultimately mental is not health at all."

East and West

With the last four limbs of Yoga—Pratyahara, Dharana, Dhyana and Samadhi—we leave the external world and enter the internal world of consciousness. This is a natural and easy transition for the Easterner, but many Westerners will stand hesitantly on the brink of what are to them uncharted waters. To understand why this is so one must consider the traditional difference between Western and Eastern thought.

Western thought has been directed outwards, concerning itself chiefly with material things. Great advances have been made in such sciences as nuclear physics, but the youngest science and the one in which least progress has been made is that which seeks to understand our own minds—psychology.

The approach of the Eastern thinker, on the other hand, has been philosophical. He has turned his thought inwards, exploring consciousness to its very source. While progress to the Westerner means faster travel, more material comforts, etc., to the Easterner it means spiritual self-unfoldment. The latter unhesitatingly leaves the external world to enter the internal world of consciousness, because he feels and believes that the two worlds are one. In entering himself he comes closer to the vast outside universe; external and internal being only relative terms.

"Make peace with yourself," says St. Isaak of Syria, "and heaven and earth will make peace with you. Endeavour to enter your own inner cell, and you will see the heavens; because the one and the other are one and the same, and when you enter one you see the two."

As long as we in the West keep turning our attention and energies outwards, there can be no possibility of inner development. The psycho-analyst Dr. C. G. Jung has said: "We have built a monumental world round about us, and have slaved for it with unequalled energy. But it is so imposing only because we have spent upon the outside all that is imposing in our natures—and what we find when we look within must necessarily be as it is, shabby and insufficient."

Not only Jung, but many other leading Western psychologists, have studied and appreciated the significance and value of Eastern psychic exploration, among them Professor William James, who said: "The most venerable system and the one whose results have the most voluminous experimental corroboration, is undoubtedly Yoga. The results claimed, and certainly in many cases accorded by impartial judges, is strength of character, personal power, unshakeability of soul."

The subconscious is a term beloved of present-day psychologists, writers and journalists. It refers to that part of our minds of which we are not consciously aware, but which nevertheless is the largest part of our minds, and influences to a powerful degree our everyday actions. The subconscious is the storehouse of our memories. Through hypnosis and psycho-analysis it can be contacted. The ancient Yogis knew about and understood the workings of the subconscious mind thousands of years ago, just as they formulated the philosophic doctrine Syadvada, which resembles relativism, two thousand years before Einstein's discovery.

The idea of meditation, which is the basis of Raja Yoga practice, is strange to the West, unlike the East where not only priests and monks and the very devout set aside time for daily meditation, but also people in all walks of life.

Dr. Lily Abegg, in her book *The Mind of East Asia*, says: "Not only priests and monks take part in the Zen exercises, but also many laymen who wish to study the methods of contemplation. In Japan, particularly during the last war, these attracted large numbers from all sections of the population. . . . Not only officers, businessmen and ministers of state, but also postal officials, shop assistants, railwaymen, young schoolboys and many others, meditated. It went so far that even in training establishments, schools and also in many factories and other concerns a short period was set aside in the mornings for 'meditation' (of course not necessarily of a Zen-Buddhist kind!)."

Can you see this happening in the West, where the craze for speed and action leaves no time for so vague and tenuous a thing as meditation? We live lives of hustle and strain, without getting to know our true Self. The Easterner looks on the Westerner as ignorant because he does not know his own nature and is not master of his soul. The Westerner looks on the Easterner as ignorant because he has made little progress in exploring nature and developing the sciences.

Dr. Lily Abegg says: "Our consciousness developed in an extravert, that of the East Asians in an introvert manner. The East Asians followed the inner way and reached a high level of consciousness relatively early; whereas in their knowledge of the world they remained far behind us. They know man better, and we are better acquainted with the world. That is how those mutual accusations of defective knowledge, which are made with complete justification by each side, come about."

Yet the differences may not be so great as we think. The latest scientific discoveries in the field of nuclear physics, for example, seem merely to corroborate what the ancient East stated in philosophic terms. No race or portion of the globe has the monopoly of wisdom. East can learn from West, and West from East. The outgoing consciousness of the Occident requires the influence of the ingoing consciousness of the Orient. The life-negation of the East requires an awakening from the life-affirmation of the West.

Levels of Consciousness

The aim of Yoga is the attainment of the super-conscious state of samadhi. To this end are the physical preparation of Hatha Yoga and the meditative practices of Raja Yoga devised. The Yogi believes that conscious evolution is inherent in all men. Each one of them possesses the power of spiritual self-unfoldment. Men live in different levels of being, from the animal to the divine. Yoga is the system whereby a man can work in his own lifetime to achieve a higher stage of consciousness.

This idea of different levels of consciousness—though an old one—will be strange to most Westerners. We are inclined to take our consciousness for granted. But is the one we know the only one possible? Does there not seem irrefutable evidence that other people experience different levels of consciousness from ourselves? And have we not had our own moments of heightened consciousness, often in childhood?

Dr. Maurice Nicoll says: "We know that there can enter into all that we see, do, think and feel, a sense of unreality. Sometimes it takes the form of seeing the unreality of other people. We observe that some force seems to be hurrying everyone to and fro. We see transiently a puppet-world, in which people are moved as by strings. Sometimes, however, in place of unreality, an extraordinary intensity of reality is felt.

We suddenly see someone for the first time, whom we have known for years, in a kind of stillness. We perceive the reality of another existence, or we perceive the existence of nature, suddenly, as a marvel, for the first time. The same experience, felt in relation to oneself, is THE SENSE OF ONE'S OWN EXISTENCE, INDEPENDENT OF EVERYTHING ELSE, the realization of one's invisibility, the perception of I, of duration without time.

"These feelings surround our natural reality. I think that they show us clearly enough that there are other meanings of oneself, or forms of conscious experience."

And William James said: "Our normal waking consciousness, rational consciousness, is but one special type of consciousness, while all about it, parted from it by the flimsiest of screens, there are potential forms of consciousness entirely different."

The Gurdjieff/Ouspensky School which has many followers in the West, says that there are seven categories of man.

Man No. 1 is Physical Man. This is animal man. He identifies his "I" with his body. The centre of gravity of his psychic life lies in the moving centre. The moving and instinctive functions constantly outweigh the emotional and thinking functions. For him knowledge is based upon imitation or instincts, learned by heart, crammed or drilled into him. He learns like a parrot.

Man No. 2 is Emotional Man. His centre of gravity

lies in the emotional centre, the emotional functions outweighing all others. He is the man of feeling, learning by likes and dislikes.

Man No. 3 is Intellectual Man, the man of reason. The centre of gravity of his psychic life is in the intellectual centre, where thinking functions are gaining the upper hand over the moving, instinctive and emotional. His knowledge is that of the bookworm.

All men, says this school, are born one of these three types of men. But by training, self-discipline and strife, higher levels of consciousness can be reached.

Man No. 4 is an intermediate stage. He has become conscious of his possible self-unfoldment. He is beginning to acquire a permanent centre of gravity. One dominant, permanent "I" is fighting to master the multiplicity of "I's" that previously struggled for possession of his mind. He is being emancipated from the subjective elements in his knowledge and is beginning to move along the path towards objective knowledge.

Man No. 5 has reached unity. His knowledge is whole, indivisible knowledge. He has one indivisible "I" and his knowledge belongs to it. What he knows the whole of him knows.

Man No. 6 differs from Man No. 7 only by the fact that some of his properties have not yet become permanent. Higher centres are at work in him. He possesses powers beyond the understanding of ordinary men.

Man No. 7 has reached the highest stage of conscious evolution. He has free-will and permanent, unchangeable "I". He has objective knowledge of ALL.

Yoga and Reason

Raja Yoga, though mystical, is based on the firm foundation of reason. That some schools of Yoga allowed themselves in the course of their long history to become clouded by superstition and magic, does not alter the truth of this basis. Great Yoga teachers like Vivekananda look on Yoga as a science, free from superstition, and based on reason, only in the final stage to transcend it. He says: "To get any reason out of the mass of incongruity we call human life, we have to transcend our reason, but we must do it scientifically, slowly, by regular practice, and we must cast off all superstition. We must take up the study of the super-conscious state just as any other science. On reason we must lay our foundation, we must follow reason as far as it leads; and when reason fails, reason itself will show us the way to the highest plane. When you hear a man say, 'I am inspired', and then talk irrationally, reject it. Why? Because these three states,—instinct, reason and super-consciousness, or the unconscious, conscious, and super-conscious states —belong to one and the same mind. There are not three minds in one man, but one state of it develops into the others. Instinct develops into reason, and reason into the transcendental consciousness; therefore not one of the states contradicts the others. Real inspiration never contradicts reason, but fulfils it. Just as you find the great prophets saying, 'I come not to destroy but to fulfil', so inspiration always comes to fulfil reason, and is in harmony with it."

Raja Yoga does not ask of you anything that is unreasonable. It does not merely theorize, but asks you to try for yourself. Only by putting the technique into practice can you experience its truth.

And if you say that you do not wish to become a mystic, but merely to gain some measure of control over an unruly mind, to enrich that mind and to find tranquillity and strength with which to face an increasingly more complex and difficult life, you will find what you seek in the concentration practices of the Royal Path.

VIII

YOGA MEDITATION

The Time

Set aside fifteen to thirty minutes daily for stilling the mind and attaining inner serenity. You will look forward to these periods. The time is not wasted as you will soon discover.

You may wish to meditate immediately after performing your Asanas and Pranayama which will prepare the mind for it. Or you may prefer or find it more convenient to allot a separate time each day.

If you meditate in the morning the inner serenity achieved will be carried into working life. Many readers will object that in the morning they are too rushed. This is often the case but can be overcome by rising earlier so as to fit in the meditation period. This should not be hurried. Give it a trial and you will see how worthwhile it is.

If you meditate before going to bed in the evening the serenity produced will ensure sleep of a high quality. If you go to sleep with worries or active thoughts on your mind you will have poor quality rest, but go to bed with a peaceful mind and you will sleep like a child and awaken wonderfully refreshed in the morning.

Except for just after meals any time of the day will do for Yoga meditation. You need not of course limit yourself to one period daily, but can have several if you wish.

It is best, though, once you have decided on a time of day, to stick to it. The habit thus formed assists meditation.

A time when I always have a meditation period is when called upon to tackle some difficult or fearful task, or when worried or under emotional stress. In the sublime peace of the stilled mind fear and grief and stress are relieved and priceless courage is gained.

The Place

Yoga meditation should be performed in a quiet place free from noise, interruptions and extremes of temperature.

It can be either outdoors or indoors. It is very pleasant to meditate outdoors in peaceful and beautiful surroundings, but weather conditions and other factors usually rule this out in our part of the world.

One place in the house should be decided upon and adhered to. It should be a clean, bright and airy room. It should be without unpleasant associations. In my book *The Art of Relaxed Living* I told the story of a man who found that he could not relax in a certain room in his house. He felt the presence of some strangely disturbing force. Going over the objects in the room one by one he finally located the trouble. It was a photograph of himself as a child. The trouble was that the photograph showed a little boy with a glorious head of curls, whereas the man was now bald.

Whatever the room you decide upon, you can make its atmosphere more conducive to meditation and relaxation by hanging pleasant paintings on the walls.

The Posture

One of the meditative postures should be used. In these seated poses the body forces are unified and gathered as in a non-leaking container. The work of the lungs and heart is made easier, the body is very still, and the spine—housing the vital nervous system—is held naturally upright.

People who because of age, or any other reason, cannot adopt even the Easy Posture (Sukhasana) should use a comfortable straight-backed chair.

As in performing Pranayama, spine and head should be kept erect and in a straight line. A wall or door may be used for support, and a cushion can be placed against the small of the back to help keep it straight. Sit on a cushion or folded rug or blanket.

If the body and neck muscles are weak the posture will not be firm and steady, a necessity for Yoga meditation. Hence the value of the preparatory Hatha Yoga exercises can be appreciated.

The body must be held perfectly still, naturally braced, yet not tensed. It must not intrude into consciousness. It is a mistake to place oneself in a painfully contorted position and expect to achieve success in stilling the mind. If sense-withdrawal (Pratyahara) is to be achieved there must be no discomfort. This seems obvious to me, but there are many fanatics who suffer in the difficult Lotus Posture (Padmasana) in the belief that it is the only way to success.

The meditative postures have been proved to be the finest positions for calming and mastering the mind, but remember that the Indian Yogi is familiar with these postures from an early age and spends hours daily thus seated. They are completely comfortable to him. He feels no strain.

If there is any strain at all make do with the Easy Posture, using a wall or door for back support, or just a chair. Many readers may wonder why lying on your back is not the best position to adopt. It is because a recumbent position would naturally tend to promote a feeling of drowsiness and this is not desirable in Yoga meditation, for in doing it you are not asleep, but rather very much awake and alert.

Curbing the Restless Mind

In the *Bhagavad Gita* we find the following quotation :

Arjuna says: "For the mind is verily restless, O Krishna; it is impetuous, strong and difficult to bend, I deem it as hard to curb as the wind."

Krishna answers: "Without doubt, O Mighty-Armed, the mind is hard to curb and restless, but it may be curbed by constant practice and by indifference."

Vivekananda says: "From our childhood upwards

we have been taught only to pay attention to things external, but never to things internal, hence most of us have nearly lost the faculty of observing the internal mechanism. To turn the mind, as it were, inside, stop it from going outside, and then to concentrate all its powers, and throw them upon the mind itself, in order that it may know its own nature, analyse itself— is very hard work. Yet that is the only way to anything which will be a scientific approach to the subject."

Yes, the mind is difficult to tame, especially if it has been allowed to run loose for many years. But it can be mastered as the *Gita* says "by constant practice".

The first step in this practice is Sense-Withdrawal, called by the Yogis Pratyahara.

Remember that Raja Yoga can only be fully understood by living it, by experiencing it for yourself; then what seemed before to be impossibly complex and incomprehensible will become clear and progress will be speeded up incredibly.

Sense-Withdrawal (Pratyahara)

Pratyahara is a detaching of the mind from the sense-organs. The word means "gathering towards". It checks the outgoing powers of the mind and turns them inwards. It is a gathering in and integration of the previously scattered mental energies. In Pratyahara one frees oneself from the thraldom of the sense-organs.

"When the senses have withdrawn from their objects and transmuted themselves into the modes of

consciousness, this is called 'the Withdrawal', Pratyahara" (*Yoga Aphorisms* of Patanjali 2, 54).

"The adept in yoga gives himself up to 'Withdrawal' and stops the traffic of the senses with their
objects which are word, sight, etc., to which they are
invariably attached. He then makes his senses work for
his Consciousness and the ever-agitated senses are
controlled. No yogi can achieve the aim of yoga
without controlling the senses."

(Vishnu Purana).

The external world is shut out in Yoga meditation.
This detaching from the sense-organs all of us do every
day. As I type this sentence, for example, I am conscious only of the idea I wish to express and of the
letters tumbling quickly on to the page. Yet now, at
the end of it, I can pause and be conscious of so much
more. The feel of the chair supporting me, the flicker-
ing of the fire whose heat reaches out across the room
towards me, birds chirping on the roof-tops outside
the house, and so on. To get things done in life we must
select our sense impressions, for we are being bom-
barded by a multiplicity of them every day. We may
not be conscious of the ticking of a clock until it stops,
then we instantly notice the fact.

The sense-organs themselves are merely the
"middle men" between the external world and consciousness. The eyes, for example, do not see in
themselves, but are merely the instrument of consciousness. The real organ of vision is in a nerve centre
of the brain. A man may be asleep with his eyes open,

yet seeing nothing. Pictures are striking the retinae of his eyes, but the man will not be aware of them, because he is not 'at home' in consciousness to do so.

Under hypnosis a person's sense-organs can come completely under the control of the hypnotist. He will tell his subject that his arm feels nothing, and true enough, when a match flame is held to it, nothing is felt. He will tell his subject that a piece of raw potato he is eating is a peach, and the distinct flavour of a peach is experienced. He can open the subject's eyes and make him see whatever he wishes him to see.

Vivekananda, in his *Raja Yoga*, warns against allowing one's mind to become controlled by others. Sense-Withdrawal is something which you must do for yourself, your "I" must be in complete control. Vivekananda says: "the faith-healers teach people to deny misery and pain and evil. Their philosophy is rather roundabout; but it is a part of Yoga upon which they have somehow stumbled. Where they succeed in making a person throw off suffering by denying it, they really use a part of Pratyahara, as they make the mind of the person strong enough to ignore the senses. The hypnotists in a similar manner, by their suggestion, excite in the patient a sort of morbid Pratyahara for the time being. The so-called hypnotic suggestion can only act upon a weak mind. And until the operator, by means of fixed gaze or otherwise, has succeeded in putting the mind of the subject in a sort of passive, morbid condition, his suggestions never work.

"Now the control of the centres which is established in a hypnotic patient or the patient of faith-healing, by the operator, for a time is reprehensible, because it leads to ultimate ruin. It is not really controlling the brain centres by the power of one's own will, but is, as it were, stunning the patient's mind for a time by sudden blows which another's will delivers to it. It is not checking by means of reins and muscular strength the mad career of a fiery team, but rather by asking another to deliver heavy blows on the heads of the horses, to stun them for a time into gentleness. . . .

"Every attempt at control which is not voluntary, not with the controller's own mind, is not only disastrous, but it defeats the end. The goal of each soul is freedom, mastery: freedom from the slavery of matter and thought, mastery of external and internal nature. Instead of leading towards that, every will-current from another, in whatever form it comes, either as direct control of organs, or as forcing to control them while under a morbid condition, only rivets one link more to the already existing heavy chain of bondage of past thoughts, past superstitions. Therefore, beware how you allow yourselves to be acted upon by others."

Raja Yoga does not teach morbid introspection or useless day-dreaming. There is all the difference in the world between these two states and Pratyahara, Dharana, Dhyana and Samadhi. If a person finds on meditating that he has dozed off or slipped into involuntary reverie, then he should know that he is

performing the exercises incorrectly and must bring
the wayward attention back to its task. The Raja
Yoga mental states are positive and alert.

Breathing

Pratyahara should be aided by quiet breathing.
When we are agitated our breathing is fast and jerky,
but if we breathe quietly and evenly tranquillity of
mind is promoted. At first you will have to do this
deliberately. As you sit motionless in a meditative
posture, inhale and exhale slowly through the nose.
Let the inhalations and exhalations be long and
controlled throughout. This form of breathing during
meditation will become a habit; you will no longer
be conscious of it, just as you should not be conscious
of your seated body.

Thought Observation and Control

The Yogi seeks to gain control over his thoughts.
He seeks the power to select those he considers to be
of value and to banish the rest.

People who may be very fussy about what they eat
will think nothing of allowing harmful thoughts to
dominate their minds.

Mason wrote: "On the whole, it is of as great
importance for a man to take heed what thoughts he
entertains, as what company he keeps; for they have
the same effect on the mind. Bad thoughts are as
infectious as bad company; and good thoughts solace,
instruct and entertain the mind, like good company.

And this is one great advantage of retirement, that a man may choose what company he pleases from within himself. . . . As in the world we oftener light into bad company than good, so in solitude we are oftener troubled with impertinent and unprofitable thoughts, than entertained with agreeable and useful ones: and a man that hath so far lost command of himself, as to lie at the mercy of every foolish or vexing thought, is much in the same situation as a host whose house is open to all comers; whom, though ever so noisy, rude, or troublesome, he cannot get rid of; but with this difference, that the latter hath some recompense for his trouble, the former none at all, but is robbed of his peace and quiet for nothing."

Resolve now that your mind will no longer be open to all comers, that you will cease to be the slave of your thoughts and desires.

Most of the thoughts that crowd our minds so persistently every day are useless. Each day try and cut down their number. There is no need for excessive will-power to do this, indeed it will only defeat our purpose. As with a wild horse, the mind can only be tamed by gentleness and patience.

Comfortably dressed, in peaceful surroundings, seat yourself in a steady, relaxed posture, and breathe quietly and evenly. Sit perfectly still and try to cut off all sense impressions from without. This is Pratyahara. Wrap yourself as it were in a blanket of silence.

Turn your attention inwards instead of outwards. Allow your thoughts to run through the mind as they please. Now *observe them attentively*. See how they pass in a never-ending stream. See how one thought leads to another, linked by association.

Be content with mere observation for a while. Feel yourself as a detached "I" observing your own thoughts just as if they are your fingers or toes or some other parts of the body. As they flow steadily past observe the uselessness of most of them, also their waywardness and lack of unity.

After a while, begin to lessen their number. Do not expect to make a big reduction at once. Do not expect to turn off the mind like an electric light at the touch of a switch. It just cannot be done . . . at first. Years of practice are required to still the mind to any great degree. Each meditation period try to have a few thoughts less. Even one thought less is a victory gained.

You will observe how successive thoughts are linked by association so that they follow immediately on the other. Separate two thoughts—even for a split second—and you will have a momentary glimpse of the inner stillness that is your goal.

Reducing the number of thoughts in this way gives control and self-mastery. It develops mind power. And thought-reducing practice should not be just for your daily meditation period or periods. Be vigilant. If at any time during the day you catch yourself entertaining worthless thoughts push them aside.

It will be something of a shock to many readers to observe to what extent their minds are their masters rather than their servants. But persist with the meditation. Keep on bringing the wayward mind back to its tasks. The mind that has become used to its chaotic freedom does not take kindly to discipline.

The Quest for the Self

Yoga meditation is designed so that the meditator may uncover his real "I", or Self. It does not require much self-observation to see that we have a multiplicity of "I's", each, as Ouspensky says, "seeking to be Caliph for an hour", One "I" makes a New Year resolution, another "I" breaks it before a week has passed. One "I" exists at the office, another in the home, a third on the golf-course, and so on.

Yet behind all these "I's" is the central "I", pure consciousness, an objective centre of gravity, from which our body, our emotions, and our very thoughts themselves, can be observed. Man, as far as we know, is the only living thing capable of this level of consciousness. The body, the feelings, the intellect itself, can be set aside as "not I" things.

"Pursue the enquiry 'Who am I?' relentlessly," advised an Indian guru, Sri Ramana Maharshi. "Analyse your entire personality. Try to find out where the I—thought begins. Go on with your meditations. Keep turning your attention within. One day the wheel of thought will slow down and an intuition will mysteriously arise. Follow that intuition, let your thinking stop and it will eventually lead you to the goal."

We have already seen that, involuntarily by hypnosis, voluntarily by Pratyahara, the sense-organs can be cut off from their centres of consciousness. A burning match applied to the back of the hand of a hypnotized person may not be felt. Some Yogis detach themselves to such an extent from their bodies that they can be buried alive, drink poison, or walk through fire, without coming to any harm. Such exhibitionistic fanaticism is deplored by genuine Yogis, but it does show the extent to which the body ceases to count with a person who is firmly established in the Self. Such a person does not feel cold or heat, pain or pleasure.

Similarly we can learn to detach ourselves from the negative emotions: anger, envy, jealousy, unjustified fear, etc. In man's early quest for survival these emotions served a life-preserving purpose, but in present-day civilized life they are in the main repressed and harmful to health and peace of mind. Anger, for example, floods the bloodstream with chemicals which mobilize the body for fight. But, except in war, one can no longer expect to destroy one's enemies physically. Also anger brushes aside reason and makes us act in ways that we may regret later. Efficient living is impossible without emotional control, and Yoga promotes just such a mastery.

Just as we can observe both body and emotions as "not I" things, so the thought-observation exercises described earlier in this chapter will enable you to experience the intellect as an instrument of the Self, and the instrument of your conscious evolution.

The non-Self is the body, senses, mind. That which perceives the non-Self is the real Self.

"The Purusha, no bigger than a thumb, is the inner Self, ever seated in the heart of man. He is known by the mind, which controls knowledge, and is perceived in the heart. They who know Him become immortal. . . .

"His hands and feet are everywhere; His eyes, heads, and faces are everywhere; His ears are everywhere; He exists compassing all.

"Himself devoid of senses, He shines through the functions of the senses. He is the capable ruler of all; He is the refuge of all; He is great. . . .

"The Self, smaller than the small, greater than the great, is hidden in the hearts of creatures. The wise, by the grace of the creator, behold the Lord, majestic and desireless, and become free from grief."

(*Svetasvatara Upanishad*, III, 13, 16, 17, 20).

Having uncovered the Self, the Yogi then seeks to experience its union with the universal Overself (Brahman).

IX

YOGA CONCENTRATION (DHARANA)

"To maintain the mind fixed on one spot is called concentration" (*Aphorisms* of Patanjali, 3, 1).

When by Pratyahara the tyranny of the senses has been checked, it becomes easier for the mind's energies to be focused on one point. This action, in Yoga, is called Dharana. Raja Yoga develops this power of concentration to an intense degree which can lead to psychic powers, though these powers are not its aim.

The power of the mind is greatest when instead of its forces being scattered they are brought together and focused on a point. This bringing to bear of the full weight of the intellect on a subject can result in intuitive knowledge or revelation. The Yogis say that many of the great Western inventors and intellectual giants of the past hit on Raja Yoga methods by accident, or actually practised them not knowing that they did so.

Dharana is another step on the path to Self-realization. Yoga writers have compared the mind to the surface of a pool, which is constantly troubled and in motion because of the agitation of our thoughts. If we can still this flow of thoughts and hold the mind steady, then pure consciousness, our inner Self, will be revealed and seen at the bottom of the pool. Patanjali says that Yoga is restraining the mind-stuff (Chitta) from taking various forms (Vrittis). The Chitta can be compared to the surface waters of a pool, and the Vrittis are the thought waves that cross it.

Aid to Successful Living

The ability to concentrate sharply to bring all your attention to the task in hand or the object of study, is one of the greatest keys to successful living. The man with highly developed powers of concentration can get through a tremendous amount of work. He can work with great efficiency. He can study with great intensity.

The great artist is lost in his work. All his attention is directed towards the canvas. All his faculties are brought to bear on the task in hand.

Concentration is one of the chief secrets of success in games and on the sports field. Watch the star footballer about to take a penalty kick, the master golfer attempting a long putt, the skilled snooker-player about to pot a critical black. All three will have one thing in common . . . intense concentration!

"Genius is concentration", said Schiller.

The concentrative energies of the mind will be aided if in daily life you give your full attention to things. Most people go through life in a sort of waking-sleep. The Yogi gives his full attention to even the smallest task, and at the same time manages to be very alive and alert. This is termed in Yoga Samprajanya or Awareness.

Concentration Exercises

The Yogi stills the mind and makes it steady by focusing it to a point just as the rays of the sun are captured and brought to a point of burning intensity by means of a magnifying glass. To achieve this feat various aids may be employed.

One of these is to focus your gaze on some object. It is best if the object is small rather than large.

If you are meditating outdoors you may choose a flower, a bush on a distant hill, a small, white cloud suspended motionless in a sky of amethyst, a stone protruding from the swirling waters of a mountain stream.

If you are indoors you may choose an ornament, a flower in a vase, an apple, perhaps a brightly shining star observed in the evening from a bedroom window. You may choose a photograph of a pleasant scene or of a loved one, or a painting of a religious subject or landscape of great beauty. You can make your own choice and try several until you find those that most appeal to you. Patanjali says in one of his Sutras that the Yogi can meditate on "anything that appeals to one as good".

Whatever object you choose it is best to focus the gaze on some central point. The attention should be directed to this spot as a torch-beam illuminates one spot in a dark room and is rested there steadily yet impalpably. If you use a portrait photograph, gaze into the eyes of the person. If you use a landscape painting, fix your gaze on a tree or some other object.

At first you will be sure to find that you cannot keep your attention on the object for very long. The mind will wander off into involuntary reverie. Suddenly, perhaps minutes later, you will "wake up" from your reverie to realize that the object of concentration has been entirely neglected. You stare at the object for a while but soon it is forgotten. You are thinking instead about what you will do tomorrow, what happened that afternoon, the show you saw last night, your job, income tax, the state of the world . . . anything but the object of concentration. Don't get angry with yourself. Don't become tensed up about it. Instead, gently coax your attention back to its task. Great force is not required in this work. Considerable effort will tire you and defeat your purpose. It is a fault if the face is screwed up and the body muscles are tensed in concentration.

Let us see an example of Yoga concentration at work, taking for our object something simple and pleasant—an apple. The technique followed here has been found by the author to give the best results.

Set the apple eighteen inches before you on the ground, or on a low stool or table. Let it be a handsome apple with a smooth, well-polished skin. If you can have a light shining on it so much the better.

Now examine the apple with all your senses. Do this slowly, thoroughly. Study the apple's appearance:

its size, shape, texture and colouring. See how when you study it closely you find that it has not just one or two colours as you thought at first, but numerous colours. There is yellow there, and green and brown and russet and red. There is a dent where it has fallen, ripened by the sun, on to the lush orchard grass. Now lift it to your face and feel its cool, smooth skin against your cheek. Touch it lightly with your lips. Smell its clear, fresh tang.

Then set it down again before you, keeping your gaze focused steadily upon it. Now start thinking about it: how it grew, how it ripened in the sun, how it dropped from the tree, how it was packed and despatched to the wholesaler who sold it to the shop where you bought it.

No superfluous thoughts must be allowed to intrude into this concentrated examination of the apple. If they do, push then gently aside and bring the attention back to its task.

Dhyana

Having exhausted all possible thoughts about the apple, the next stage is no longer to think about the size, shape, texture, colouring, smell, feel or history of the apple, but to fix in the mind the single idea *apple*, the essence as it were distilled from the previous few minutes' thought. With the eyes still fixed steadily on the apple, hold the idea *apple* unwaveringly in the mind. This is Dharana proper. Hold it for some time and you will attain the next Yoga limb, Dhyana, which if maintained for several minutes can lead to Samadhi, when the perceiver and the thing perceived have become one.

When the mind's energies are focused on a selected point and held there, so that but one thought wave, steady and straight, disturbs the surface of the mind-stuff (Chitta), this is called Contemplation (Dhyana). When Contemplation is maintained for some time, even this one remaining wave fades away and the untroubled, mindless superconscious state of Samadhi ensues.

Visualization

Up to now we have been dealing with Dharana practised with the eyes open so as to fix the gaze on some object; later you should concentrate with the eyes closed. This banishes external sense-impressions, making Pratyahara and the one-pointing of the mind easier. The object should then be held before the mind's eye.

Most people can with a little practice acquire the necessary powers of visualization. We each possess within us a private mental cinema on whose screens we project our hopes, fears and memories. Without having to travel to a well-loved beauty spot, and without spending a single penny, a person with strongly developed powers of visualization is able to transport himself to that place and see it clearly before his inner eye. He can see it in detail and in colour, and if his imagination is lively he will hear the sounds appropriate to the scene, the singing of birds or the sound of the wind or the sea.

The development of such powers of visualization is well worthwhile, apart from its use in Raja Yoga. It means you can store up a private collection of pictures which can be enjoyed at any time. Scenes of great beauty which you witnessed on your holidays, the look on the face of a child or a loved one . . . all these need not be lost in the maw of devouring time, but captured and filed away in your mental projection room for the rest of your life.

Still using an apple for our example as the object of concentration, the meditator may study it intently for a while, then close his eyes and still picture the apple, clearly showing behind the closed lids. After some practice at this the actual apple may be dispensed with and only its inner reflection used. The same applies to any other objects you may use for Dharana.

The devout Christian may wish to concentrate on a vision of Lord Jesus or the Virgin Mary, the devout Hindu on the face of Lord Krishna, and so on.

Many Yogis fix their inner gaze on the space between the eyebrows, or some other part of the body.

In the *Bhagavad-Gita* we find:

"Shutting out the external contact with sense-objects, the eyes fixed between the eyebrows, and equalizing the currents of Prana (incoming breath) and Apana (the outgoing breath) inside the nostrils, the meditative man, having mastered the senses, mind and intellect, being freed from desire, fear and anger, and regarding freedom as his supreme goal, is liberated forever."

In Dharana, consciousness can be directed to any part of the body. If you think of a spot on the palm of your hand and concentrate intensely on it for some time, it will begin to redden and burn just as if the rays of the sun were being focused there by a magnifying glass. The powers of the mind are developed to such an extent by adepts that even the sympathetic nervous system comes under the control of the will. They can control the beating of the heart, for example. This has been authentically proved many times. The advanced Yogi is able to direct his consciousness to any part of his body, external or internal, and hold it there.

The Mystic Sounds (Nadas)

Sounds also may be used to hold the attention. You can concentrate on the ticking of a watch in a quiet room; or, if outdoors, you can close your eyes and listen to the sound of a waterfall or stream.

Some gurus instruct their pupils in the art of concentrating on inner sounds (nadas). The ears are closed with the fingers and the attention is focused on the sounds to be heard. By practice the mind is able to hold on to the finer and subtler sounds, until eventually liberation is achieved.

Here is the *Hatha Yoga Pradipika's* instructions on listening to the nadas:

"The sound which a muni (sage) hears by closing

his ears with his fingers should be heard attentively, till the mind becomes steady in it. By practising with this nada, all other external sounds are stopped. The Yogi becomes happy by overcoming all distractions within fifteen days. In the beginning, the sounds heard are of a great variety and very loud; but as the practice increases, they become more and more subtle. In the first stage, the sounds are surging, thundering like the beating of kettledrums, and jingling ones. In the intermediate stage, they are like those produced by conch, Mridanga, bells, etc. In the last stage, the sounds resemble those from tinklets, flute, Vina, bee, etc. These various kinds of sounds are heard as being produced in the body. Though hearing loud sounds like those of thunder, kettledrums, etc., one should try to get in touch with subtler sounds only. Leaving the loudest, taking up the subtle one, and leaving the subtle one, taking up the loudest, thus practising, the distracted mind does not wander elsewhere.

"Wherever the mind attaches itself first, it becomes steady there; and then it becomes absorbed in it. Just as a bee, drinking sweet juice, does not care for the smell of the flower; so the mind, absorbed in the nada, does not desire the object of enjoyment. The mind, like an elephant, habituated to wander in the garden of enjoyments, is capable of being controlled by the sharp goad of anahata nada (heart sound). The mind, captivated in the snare of nada, gives up all its activity; and, like a bird with clipped wings, becomes calm at once. Those desirous of the kingdom of Yoga, should take up the practice of hearing the anahata nada, with mind collected and free from all cares."

Contemplation of the Void

This is described by the *Siva Samhita* as a practice sure to bring Self-realization.

"Let him (the Yogi) contemplate on his own reflection in the sky as beyond the Cosmic Egg: in the manner previously described. Through that let him think on the Great Void unceasingly. The Great Void, whose beginning is void, whose middle is void, whose end is void, has brilliancy of tens of millions of suns, and the coolness of tens of millions of moons. By contemplating continually on this, one obtains success. Let him practise with energy daily this dhyana, within a year he shall obtain all success undoubtedly. He whose mind is absorbed in that place even for a second, is certainly a Yogi, and a good devotee, and is revered in all worlds. All his stores of sins are at once verily destroyed. By seeing it one never returns to the path of this mortal universe; let the Yogi, therefore, practise this with great care by the path of Svadhish-thana. I cannot describe the grandeur of this contem-plation. He who practises, knows."

Contemplation of the Inner Light

Patanjali gives as one of the things to be meditated upon, "The Effulgent Light".

In Samadhi a great white light may be seen, the

colourless light of pure consciousness. Sitting in a meditative posture, perfectly still, with eyes closed and senses withdrawn, the Yogi may concentrate until perceiving a small point of light before the mind's eye. By concentrating the mind's energies on it, it will grow until he becomes filled with it and Superconsciousness occurs.

A Tibetan Technique

Some Yogis use a meditative technique in which the mental image of a flower, tree or person is held for a time, then gradually demolished, bit by bit, until only a clear light remains. This technique is described in *The Tibetan Book of the Dead*, edited by Evans-Wentz.

"Whosoever thy tutelary deity may be, meditate upon the form for much time—as being apparent, yet non-existent in reality, like a form produced by a magician . . . Then let the vision of the tutelary deity melt away from the extremities, until nothing at all remaineth visible of it; and put thyself in the state of the Clearness and the Voidness—which thou canst not conceive as something—and abide in that state for a little while. Again meditate upon the tutelary deity; again meditate upon the Clear Light; do this alternately. Afterwards allow thine own intellect to melt away gradually, beginning from the extremities."

Blotting out the Ego

A similar technique requires the meditator to feel

his closed eyes and his head to be filled with foaming water. Next he must meditate on his body from the throat to the stomach, filling it with imaginary water. Then he mentally fills all of his body, including the arms and legs, with cool water, the colour of glass. After he has filled all of himself with pure water, he should imagine that the room too is filled with it. When this has been clearly experienced, he must gradually drain away the water, reversing the previous process. That is to say, he drains the water from the room slowly and steadily until none remains between ceiling and floor; then from his arms, legs and stomach; next from his chest and throat; finally from his head and eyes. In this way the false Ego vanishes.

A World of Diamonds

In yet another method to achieve withdrawal and onepointedness, the meditator imagines that he has a diamond in each ear, and a canopy of diamonds about his head, and that all his surroundings, whether outdoors or indoors, have been turned into diamonds (or crystal), bright, pure, clear and shutting out all sound.

Japa

In Mantra Yoga the mind is concentrated by means of Japa, the repetition of sacred syllables, words and prayers (mantras). The Japa may be voiced (vachika), whispered (upanshu), or mental (manasa), the last being considered the highest.

The sacred syllable OM (AUM) is considered the finest mantra. The Upanishads describe it as being a symbol of the whole universe and "all that is past, present, and future . . . and whatever else there is, beyond the threefold division of time."

"Meditate on Atman as AUM"; "AUM, this word, is Brahman." *Taittirya Upanishad.*

Aum is considered to be the basis of all sound— the a is formed far back in the throat, the u carries the tone forward, and the word leaves the mouth from the closed vibrating lips. Its vibrations are said to be beneficial to health and the disciplining of the mind.

Other mantras frequently used are Soham (He is I), and Hansah (I am He).

X

PSYCHIC POWERS

Samyama

The last three limbs of Yoga—Dharana, Dhyana, and Samadhi—practised together with regard to one object, are called Samyama. By making Samyama on various things intuition and advanced psychic powers are claimed by Yoga. Patanjali gives thirty-seven of these—expressed in symbolical language—but warns that these powers, if taken up for worldly ends, are dangerous and obstacles to Self-realization. The acquisition of psychic powers could so easily intensify Egoism, whereas the Yogi seeks to annihilate it.

The third part of Patanjali's *Yoga Aphorisms* is given to special powers resulting from the application of Samyama to certain things. I give them here in Vivekananda's translation, but without his commentaries. Readers wishing to go further into this subject should therefore obtain Vivekananda's book, or some of the other translations and commentaries.

The Thirty-Seven Psychic Powers

(1). By making Samyana on the three sorts of changes (form, time, and state) comes the knowledge of past and future.

(2). By making Samyama on word, meaning, and knowledge, which are ordinarily confused, comes the knowledge of all animal sounds.

(3). By perceiving the impressions, (comes) the knowledge of past life.

(4). By making Samyama on the signs in another's body, knowledge of his mind comes.

(5). But not its contents, that not being the object of the Samyama.

(6). By making Samyama on the form of the body, the perceptibility of the form being obstructed, and the power of manifestation in the eye being separated, the Yogi's body becomes unseen.

(7). By this the disappearance or concealment of words which are being spoken, and such other things, are also explained.

(8). Karma is of two kinds, soon to be fructified, and late to be fructified. By making Samyama on these, or by the signs called Arishta, portents, the Yogis know the exact time of separation from their bodies.

(9). By making Samyama on friendship, mercy, etc., the Yogi excels in the respective qualities.

(10). By making Samyama on the strength of the elephant and others, their respective strength comes to the Yogi.

(11). By making Samyama on the Effulgent Light comes the knowledge of the fine, the obstructed, and the remote.

(12). By making Samyama on the sun, (comes) the knowledge of the world.

(13). On the moon, (comes) the knowledge of the cluster of stars.

(14). On the pole-star, (comes) the knowledge of the motions of the stars.

(15). On the navel circle, (comes) the knowledge of the constitution of the body.

(16). On the hollow of the throat, (comes) cessation of hunger.

(17). On the nerve called Kurma, (comes) fixity of the body.

(18). On the light emanating from the top of the head, sight of the Siddhas.

(19). Or by the power of Pratibha, all knowledge.

(20). In the heart, knowledge of minds.

(21). Enjoyment comes by the non-discrimination of the soul and Sattva which are totally different. The latter whose actions are for another is separate from the self-centred one. Samyama on the self-centred one gives knowledge of the Purusha.

(22). From that arises the knowledge belonging to Pratibha and (supernatural) hearing, touching, seeing, tasting, and smelling.

Here Patanjali interjects a warning :

These are obstacles to Samadhi: but they are powers in the worldly state.

(23). When the cause of bondage of the Chitta has become loosened, the Yogi, by his knowledge of its channels of activity (the nerves), enters another's body.

(24). By conquering the current called Udana the Yogi does not sink in water, in swamps, he can walk on thorns, etc., and can die at will.

(25). By the conquest of the current Samana he is surrounded by a blaze of light.

(26). By making Samyama on the relation between the ear and the Akasha (ether) comes divine hearing.

(27). By making Samyama on the relation between the Akasha and the body and becoming light as cotton, wool, etc., through meditation on them, the Yogi goes through the skies.

(28). By making Samyama on the "real modifications" of the mind, outside of the body, called great disembodiedness, comes disappearance of the covering to light.

(29). By making Samyama on the gross and fine forms of the elements, their essential traits, the inherence of the Gunas in them and on their contributing to the experience of the soul, comes mastery of the elements.

(30). From that comes minuteness, and the rest of the powers, "glorification of the body", and indestructibleness of the bodily qualities.

The "glorification of the body" is beauty, complexion, strength, adamantine hardness.

Minuteness and the rest of the powers here referred to are the eight attainments, said also to result from the Hatha Yoga practice of Pranayama. They are:

(1). Anima.   To become as small as an atom.
(2). Mahima.   To become very large.
(3). Laghima.   To become very light.
(4). Garima.   To become very heavy.
(5). Prapti.   To be able to go anywhere.
(6). Prakamya.   To have one's desires fulfilled.
(7). Vashitva. To control all nature.
(8). Ishitva.   To possess the power to create.

(31). By making Samyama on the objectivity and power of illumination of the organs, on egoism, the inherence of the Gunas in them, and on their contributing to the experience of the soul, comes the conquest of the organs.

(32). From that comes to the body the power and rapid movement like the mind, power of the organs independently of the body, and the conquest of nature.

(33). By making Samyama on the discrimination between the Sattva and the Purusha come omnipotence and omniscience.

(34). By giving up even these powers comes the destruction of the very seed of evil, which leads to Kaivalya (isolation).

(35). By making Samyama on a particle of time and its precession and succession comes discrimination.

(36). The saving knowledge is that knowledge of discrimination which simultaneously covers all objects, in all their variations.

(37). By the similarity of purity between the Sattva and the Purusha comes Kaivalya.

In Chapter I, 35 of his *Yoga Aphorisms* Patanjali says: "Those forms of concentration that bring extraordinary sense-perceptions cause perseverance of the mind."

And Vivekananda comments:

"This naturally comes with Dharana, concentration; the Yogis say, if the mind becomes concentrated on the tip of the nose, one begins to smell, after a few days, wonderful perfumes. If it becomes concentrated at the root of the tongue, one begins to hear sounds; if on the tip of the tongue, one begins to taste wonderful flavours; if on the middle of the tongue, one feels as if he were coming in contact with something. If one concentrates his mind on the palate he begins to see peculiar things. If a man whose mind is disturbed wants to take up some of these practices of Yoga, yet doubts the truth of them, he will have his doubts set at rest when, after a little practice, these things come to him, and he will persevere."

Compare this with the *Siva Samhita:*

"Let the Yogi seat himself in the Padmasana and fix his attention on the cavity of the throat, let him place his tongue at the base of the palate; by this he will extinguish hunger and thirst. Below the cavity of the throat, there is a beautiful Nadi (vessel) called Kurma; when the Yogi fixes his attention on it, he acquires great concentration of the thinking principle.

When the Yogi constantly thinks that he has got a third eye—the eye of Siva—in the middle of his forehead, he then perceives a fire brilliant like lightning. By contemplating on this light, all sins are destroyed, and even the most wicked person obtains the highest end. If the experienced Yogi thinks of this light day and night he sees Siddhas (adepts), and can certainly converse with them. He who contemplates on Sunya (the void), while walking or standing, dreaming or waking, becomes altogether ethereal and is absorbed in the Chid Akasa. The Yogi, desirous of success, should always obtain this knowledge; by habitual exercise he becomes equal to me; through the force of this knowledge he becomes the beloved of all. Having conquered all the elements and being void of all hopes and worldly connections, when the Yogi sitting in the Padmasana, fixes his gaze on the tip of his nose, his mind becomes dead and he obtains the spiritual power called Khecari. The great Yogi beholds light, pure as holy mountain, and through the force of his exercise in it, he becomes the lord and guardian of the light. Stretching himself on the ground, let him contemplate on this light; by so doing all his weariness and fatigue are destroyed. By contemplating on the back part of his head, he becomes the conqueror of death."

Kundalini Yoga

The Laya (Latent) School of Yoga, by concentrating on seven main centres, or chakras, situated between the base of the spine and the brain, attain superconsciousness by arousing what is symbolically termed "the coiled serpent" Kundalini, said to be asleep in the first or root centre at the base of the spine. It is described by some writers as electricity, a negative pole being freed and racing up to unite with the positive pole in the brain. This power when aroused, can be passed up the centre of the spine, from chakra to chakra, until it reaches the top of the head, when superconsciousness is achieved. Great psychic powers are said to result from this Yoga, but readers should be warned that it could be dangerous unless practised under a guru or Yoga master.

The Kundalini passes upwards through a channel situated in the centre of the spine and called the Sushumna-Nadi. Two other Nadi run alongside it, the negative Ida-Nudi on its left, and the positive Pingala-Nadi on its right. Investigators state that the Yoga chakras are approximate with centres of bunched nerve ganglia in the body; others approximate the chakras with the chief bodily glands. The Yogis have named each centre and the awakening of Kundalini is assisted by visualizing the chakras as coloured lotus flowers.

THE CHAKRAS

(1). The Root Centre (Muladhara). Situated just above the anus, at the very base of the spine. It is here that the coiled energy lies sleeping.

(2). The Support of the Life Breath Centre (Svadhishthana). Situated in the genital area.

(3). The Jewel City Centre (Manipura). Situated in the region of the navel.

(4). The Unstruck Sound Centre (Anahata). Situated in the heart.

(5). The Great Purity Centre (Vishuddha). Situated in the throat.

(6). The Command Centre (Ajna). Situated in the middle of the brow.

(7). The Thousand Petalled Lotus Centre (Sahasrara). At the crown of the skull. The centre of Self-realization.

There are several secondary chakras: Lalana, situated between the Vishuddha and Ajna centres; Brahmarandhra, situated just above the Ajna centre; Manas, close to the Ajna centre; Soma, just above the Manas chakra; Karanarupa, a group of "seven casual forms" situated near the Ajna centre; and Manipitha, situated above the "seven casual forms".

XI

SELF-REALIZATION (SAMADHI)

Samadhi: With and Without Seed

"When alone the object of contemplation remains and one's own form is annihilated, this is known as Samadhi" (*Aphorisms* of Patanjali 3, 3).

There are two stages of Samadhi, described as with-seed and the seedless. The second stage comes when even the idea of control is absent, having faded away. If we think of our mind as a pool and of thoughts as the waves that cross its surface, then Dharana reduces all waves to a single one; Dhyana maintains it fixed for some minutes at a stretch, and with Samadhi with-seed the wave is reduced to the gentle one that is the thought of control itself. When even this wave fades away, advanced Samadhi has been achieved.

Vivekananda explains it:

"You remember that our goal is to perceive the Soul Itself. We cannot perceive the Soul because It has got mingled up with nature, with the mind, with the body. The ignorant man thinks his body is the Soul. The learned man thinks his mind is the Soul; but both of them are mistaken. What makes the Soul get mingled up with all this? Different waves in the

Chitta rise and cover the Soul; we only see a little reflection of the Soul through these waves. So, if the wave is one of anger, we see the Soul as angry; 'I am angry,' one says. If it is one of love, we see ourselves reflected in that wave, and say we are loving. If that wave is one of weakness, and the Soul is reflected in it, we think we are weak. These various ideas come from these impressions, these Samskaras covering the Soul. The real nature of the Soul is not perceived as long as there is one single wave in the lake of the Chitta; this real nature will never be perceived until all the waves have subsided; so, first, Patanjali teaches us the meaning of these waves; secondly, the best way to repress them; and thirdly, how to make one wave so strong as to suppress all other waves, fire eating fire as it were. When only one remains, it will be easy to suppress that also; and when that is gone, this Samadhi or concentration is called seedless. It leaves nothing, and the Soul is manifested just as It is, in Its own glory."

Later (in *Raja Yoga*) he says:

". . . in this first state of Samadhi (Samadhi with seed) the modifications of the mind have been controlled, but not perfectly, because if they were, there would be no modifications. If there is a modification which impels the mind to rush out through the senses, and the Yogi tries to control it, that very control itself will be a modification. One wave will be checked by another wave, so it will not be real Samadhi, in which all the waves subside, as control itself will be a wave. Yet this lower Samadhi is very much nearer to the higher Samadhi than when the mind comes bubbling out."

This same distinction is found in Zen-Buddhist meditation, where you have the two stages of "present-heart" (Ushin) and "no-heart" (Mushin), heart here meaning consciousness.

The Zen-Buddhist, Daisetz Suzuki says :

"If you are possessed by certain thoughts, then your heart is to that extent closed to other thoughts. If you are occupied, then you can neither hear nor see anything, but if you keep your heart empty, that is to say open, then you can take in everything which approaches you—that is what is called Mushin. If, however, you are only concerned with keeping your heart empty, this very condition of your heart will prevent you from realizing Mushin or the original heart. Herein lies the difficulty of attaining the state of no-heart. But when your practising reaches maturity it comes about of its own accord. You cannot hasten this state of Mushin. As an old poem has it: 'Being mindful of not-thinking is thinking nevertheless. O that I were now beyond thinking and non-thinking.'"

Samadhi: Its Nature

To the Yogi the Postures (Asanas), Breathing Exercises (Pranayama), Sense-withdrawal (Pratyahara) Concentration (Dharana), and Contemplation (Dhyana) are but steps in a journey up a mountainside.

Raja Yoga provided the final moves to the pinnacle of supreme bliss . . . Samadhi.

What is this Samadhi so earnestly sought?

It is given many names: Union, Integration, Identification, Liberation, Superconsciousness, Self-realization. It is an inner peace in whose radiance one can bask. It is above and beyond the senses. Words, therefore, cannot adequately describe it. It must be experienced.

At the point where Samadhi is reached the Ego ceases to exist. All sense of "I" and "mine-ness" is banished. It is a liberation from the tyranny of desires, fears, worries, persons, places and things.

Note this description of Ramakrishna attaining the culminating stage of Norvikalpa Samadhi: "The Universe was extinguished. Space itself was no more. At first the shadows of ideas floated in the obscure depths of the mind. Monotonously a feeble conscious-ness of the Ego went on ticking. Then that stopped too. Nothing remained but existence. The soul was lost in Self. Dualism was blotted out. Finite and infinite space were as one. Beyond word, beyond thought, he attained Brahman."

You will appreciate this better if you think of those moments in your life when you experienced the most sublime happiness. Am I not right in thinking that they were those moments when the Ego was annihilated, when you were "carried out of yourself" by an emotional experience, the sight of a glorious sunset or landscape, the sound of glorious music, a moment of truth?

The poet Tennyson spoke of: "A kind of waking trance I have frequently had, quite up from boyhood, when I have been all alone. This has generally come upon me through repeating my own name two or three times to myself, silently, till all at once, as it were, out of the intensity of consciousness of individuality, the individuality itself seemed to fade away into boundless being, and this not a confused state, but the clearest of the clearest, the surest of the surest, utterly beyond words, where death was almost a laughable impossibility, the loss of personality (if so it were) seeming no extinction but the only true life . . . I am ashamed of my feeble description. Have I not said that the state is beyond words?"

Those readers who have cultivated a love of beautiful things will understand what is meant. Those who appreciate good music will understand what is meant.

Perhaps in the language of music and the arts the voice of Superconsciousness can be heard. J. W. N. Sullivan stated that great composers like Beethoven were able in their music "to communicate valuable spiritual states which testify to the depth of the artist's nature and to the quality of his experience of life."

Music can elevate the spirit and blot out the Ego. Observe an audience held spell-bound by great music. Note how still they are, how relaxed, how steady their gaze on conductor, singer or performer.

Music lovers will know that there is often experienced a sudden upsurge of elation at certain moments in their favourite works.

Often when I have the house to myself I switch off all lights, make myself comfortable before the fire in a meditative posture, and play some records.

One of my favourites is "Death of a Novice" (La Mort De L'Escola), sung unaccompanied in Catalan by the Orfeo Catala de Barcelona.

In this amazing record the voices range from the purest boy-soprano to the most profound and deepest of bassos. These latter imitate the tolling of the funeral bell.

There is a point near the end of the work when the voices are suddenly quiet. There is a pause, a silence, then a boy-soprano commences to sing in a voice of pure silver, a shaft of radiant light that suddenly stabs into the semi-darkness of the cathedral.

At that moment I always experience a rapid outgoing of fear, desire, worry and egoism, with a resultant relaxation and inrush of an ineffable peace. There is Samadhi—perhaps only for a second—but a second of such richness as to be beyond time or measurement.

With Samadhi we enter a region of feeling, of being, where attempts at description in the rational terms of our language must necessarily be inadequate. We have the evidence of those who have experienced it that it is "beyond words". Nevertheless C. F. Morel makes a praiseworthy attempt at an explanation in rational terms: "Consciousness is . . . something intensely mobile. When the exterior world has disappeared, the circle of consciousness contracts and seems to withdraw entirely into some unknown and usually ignored cortical centre. Consciousness seems to gather itself together, to confine itself within some unknown psychic pineal gland and to withdraw into a kind of centre wherein all organic functions and all psychic forces meet, and there it enjoys unity." And Theos Bernard assures us that it "is not an imaginary or mythical state, though it is explained by myths, but is an actual condition that can be subjectively experienced and objectively observed."

Mouni Sadhu, in his *In Days of Great Peace*, (Allen and Unwin Ltd.), says that Samadhi has three phases:

"*The First*—when we feel it is approaching. In this state we can still move and talk as usual. We can compare it to early twilight before sunrise.

"*The Second* can be compared to the midday when the sun stands high in the sky. Then the mental and physical functions decline, they become dreamy, and *reality* alone, independent of all form and condition, dawns upon and illumines our being. We then *know Who we are*, we do not identify ourselves any more with our personalities, we are above and beyond them. We breathe freedom, bliss and wisdom.

"*The Third*—which comes immediately after our 'coming back' from Samadhi, is like the second twilight, this time preceding 'sunset'. We still feel in ourselves its last rays, we still clearly remember the *light*, but its vivid reality gradually fades away when we return to our 'normal' consciousness, the 'waking' state. But the remembrance of Samadhi is not completely lost. We are still unable to stay in it permanently, due to our imperfect spiritual development, but henceforth we *know* irrefutably that this state exists, that it *is* in truth, the only reality. After experiencing Samadhi even once we are different beings."

Those who have achieved mystical enlightenment are agreed on several things: Samadhi is a positive and not a negative state like sleep or hypnotic trance; and it is distinguished by two features—an altered conception of time, and the experiencing on a level of being of the unity of all life.

Living in the Now

When the mind is stilled by Raja Yoga, time—that is to say, *psychological* time—ceases to exist. For time is relative. It only exists when one thing is taken in relation to another. If I go on a train journey my leaving the train at my destination, taken in relation to my getting in, shows a passage of time. Similarly, if I think of "fruit", and in a split second follow with another thought "apples", time has passed, and I am aware of its passing. But if the mind takes one thought and holds it, one-pointed and still, time is erased, it ceases—psychologically—to exist.

In the hurly-burly of civilized living we rarely find time, or even give a thought to living in the NOW. We spend our NOW in thinking of the past or dreaming of the future. Raja Yoga enables us to be still and experience eternity, as defined by Boethius: "to hold and possess the whole fullness of life in one moment, here and now, past and present and to come."

"No reveries, no conversations, no tracing out of the meaning of phantasies, contain this *now*, which belongs to a higher order of consciousness," writes Dr. Maurice Nicoll, in his *Living Time and the Integration of the Life*. "The *time-man* in us does not know *now*. He is always preparing something in the future, or busy with what happened in the past. He is always wondering what to do, what to say, what to wear, what to eat, etc. He anticipates; and we, following him, come to the expected moment, and lo, he is already elsewhere, planning further ahead. This is *becoming*—where nothing ever *is*. We must come to our senses to begin to feel *now*. We can only feel *now* by checking this time-man, who thinks of existence in his own way. NOW enters us with a sense of something greater than passing time. NOW contains all time, all the life, and the aeon of the life. NOW is the sense of higher space. It is not the decisions of the man in time that count here, for they do not spring from NOW. All decisions that belong to the life in time, to success, to business, comfort, are about 'tomorrow'. All decisions about the right thing to do, about how to act, are about tomorrow. It is only what is done in NOW that counts, and this is a decision always about ONESELF and WITH oneself, even although its effect may touch other people's lives 'tomorrow'. NOW is spiritual. It is a state of the spirit, when it is above the stream of time-associations. Spiritual values have nothing to do with time. They are not in time, and their growth is not a matter of time. To retain the impression of their truth we must fight with time, with every notion that they belong to time, and that the passage of days will increase them. For then it will be easy for us to think it is TOO LATE, to make the favourite excuse of passing time.

"The feeling of NOW is the feeling of certainty. In NOW passing time halts, and in this halting of time one's understanding has power over one. One knows, sees, feels in oneself, apart from all outer things; and above all, one IS. . . . All insight, all revelation, all illumination, all love, all that is genuine, all that is real, lies in NOW—and in the attempt to create *now* we approach the inner precincts, the holiest part of life. For in time all things are seeking completion, but in *now* all things are complete."

Unity

To the Yogi Samadhi is the merging of the individual Soul or Self with the universal Soul or Overself.

In the *Shiva Sanhita* we find:

"As space pervades a jar both in and out, similarly within and beyond this ever-changing universe there exists one Universal Spirit.

"Having renounced all false desires and chains, the sannyasi and Yogi see certainly in their own spirit the Universal Spirit.

"Having seen the spirit that brings forth happiness in their own spirit, they forget this universe, and enjoy the ineffable bliss of Samadhi."

"Thou art that." One of the favourite spiritual meditations given by gurus to their pupils is contained in these three words. Their meaning is illustrated in this duologue from the *Chandogya Upanishad*:

"When Svetaketu was twelve years old he was sent to a teacher, with whom he studied until he was twenty-four. After learning all the Vedas, he returned home full of conceit in the belief that he was consummately well educated, and very censorious.

"His father said to him, 'Svetaketu, my child, you who are so full of your learning, and so censorious, have you asked of that knowledge by which we hear the unhearable, by which we perceive what cannot be perceived, and know what cannot be known?'

" 'What is that knowledge, sir?' asked Svetaketu.

"His father replied, 'As by knowing one lump of clay all that is made of clay is known, the difference being only in name, but the truth being that all is clay—so, my child, is that knowledge, knowing which we know all.'

" 'But surely these venerable teachers of mine are ignorant of this knowledge; for if they possessed it they would have imparted it to me. Do you, sir, therefore give me that knowledge.'

" 'So be it,' said the father . . . And he said, 'Bring me a fruit of the nyagrodha tree.'

" 'Here is one, sir.'

" 'Break it.'

" 'It is broken, sir.'

" 'What do you see there?'

" 'Some seeds, sir, exceedingly small.'

" 'Break one of these.'

" 'It is broken, sir.'

" 'What do you see there?'

" 'Nothing at all.'

"The father said, 'My son, that subtle essence which you do not perceive there—in that very essence stands the being of the huge nyagrodha tree. In that which is the subtle essence all that exists has its self. That is the True, that is the Self, and thou, Svetaketu, art That.'

" 'Pray, sir,' said the son, 'tell me more.'

" 'Be it so, my child,' the father replied; and he said, 'Place this salt in water, and come to me to-morrow morning.'

"The son did as he was told.

"Next morning, the father said, 'Bring me the salt which you put in the water.'

"The son looked for it, but could not find it; for the salt, of course, had dissolved.

"The father said, 'Taste some of the water from the surface of the vessel. How is it?'

" 'Salty.'

" 'Taste some from the middle. How is it?'

" 'Salty'.

" 'Taste some from the bottom. How is it?'

" 'Salty.'

"The father said, 'Throw the water away and then come back to me again.'

"The son did so; but the salt was not lost, for the salt exists forever.

"Then the father said, 'Here likewise in this body of yours, my son, you do not perceive the True; but there in fact it is. In that which is the subtle essence, all that exists has its self. That is the True, that is the Self, and thou, Svetaketu, art That.' "

Unity, completeness, wholeness, integration—this is the goal of all esoteric teaching; and those who work to attain the highest levels of consciousness can experience the universe as the unity its name implies.

Indeed, Western science is coming more and more to provide evidence of a physical basis for the intuitive knowledge of the Eastern mystic.

"Separate, individual existences are illusions of common sense," says Aldous Huxley, in *Ends and Means*. "Scientific investigation reveals—and these findings, as we shall see later on, are confirmed by the direct intuition of the trained mystic and contemplative—that concrete reality consists of the interdependent parts of a totality and that independent existences are merely abstractions from that reality." And later: "More recently investigators, trained in the discipline of mathematical physics and equipped with instruments of precision, have made observations from which it could be inferred that all the apparently independent existences in the world are built up of a limited number of patterns of identical units of energy. An ultimate physical identity underlines the apparent physical diversity of the world. Moreover, all apparently independent existences are in fact interdependent. Meanwhile the mystics had shown that investigators, trained in the discipline of recollection and meditation, could obtain direct experience of a spiritual unity underlying the apparent diversity of independent consciousness. They made it clear that what seemed to be the ultimate fact of personality was in reality not an ultimate fact, and that it was possible for individuals to transcend the limitations of personality and to merge their private consciousness into a greater, impersonal consciousness underlying the personal mind."

What Huxley says is borne out by the interesting report of the Peckham biologists:

". . . plant, animal and man live by the same biological law. The laws that govern growth and development apply equally to the organism as a whole, or to its parts. . . . the process of diversification so characteristic of organism and, as a result of the life process, equally apparent in the environment, must denote some PROGRESSIVE ORDER in the latter. Can it be that the environment, also 'in process', is taking on an orientation as ordered as that which the embryologist can follow so clearly in the differentiation of the embryo—like the chick developing from the amorphous material of the egg? Is, then, the process we call 'evolution', with all its manifest expressions, but one universal expression of the 'organization' of the environment itself? Is the environment ALIVE?

"The mutual action of organism and environment, associated as we rise in the biological scale with an increasing degree of autonomy of the organism, recalls forcibly to mind the circumstances of a single cell, such for instance as the liver cell, set in the body of which it is an infinitesimal part. The cell acts as liver cell carrying on the specific function of 'liverness', yet always, in health, 'aware' of, and subject to, the wider needs of the body of which it is part and from which it derives sustenance. It is the RELATIONSHIP TO THE BODY which alone gives significance to its individuality as liver cell as well as to its unique function of liverness.

"The pathologist is only too familiar with the situation that arises where this delicately poised relationship of the cell's autonomy within the sphere of a greater organization—the body—is absent. When the cell multiplies without reference to the impulses of the greater organization of the body of its inhabitation, the result is cancer, the definition of which might be stated as 'multiplication without function'—loss of individuality. Such procedure ushers in antagonism, disrupting the mutual association between the cell and its environment—and ends in the ultimate destruction of the cell, of the body in which it grows, or of both.

"Thus the body as an organization is, in fact, the ultimate significance of the cell. Can it then be that Man himself is but a cell in the body of Cosmos; and that Cosmos is organismal as he is?

"Without being able to define the factual basis of their intuition—for that can only come through science—wise men in all ages have acted with a deep intuitive consciousness of this as truth. Upon it they have built their hopes, their conduct and their religions. Only now, as intuitive apprehension seems to be wearing thin and threadbare, are men of science being led, through the study of function, to suspect that there may even be a physical basis for these primitive intuitive actions; that in fact the significance of human living lies in the degree of MUTUALITY established with an all pervading order, Nature—whether we deify her or not."

Here we have Western scientists reporting that indeed man may be—as the Eastern Yogi says— microcosm in macrocosm.

With the feeling of oneness with all life that Raja Yoga promotes comes an awakening of reverence for life and love towards all living things. Each Self is but a drop in the ocean of Overself. The Yogi realizes his brotherhood with all men. He realizes that the truth is many-sided and is therefore tolerant of the ideas and beliefs of others.

He knows the secret of happiness, which is non-

attachment to desires. For there can be no end to
desires. If they are frustrated, you feel pain and un-
happiness. If they are partly satisfied, you crave full
satisfaction. If they are fully satisfied, the desires
transfer elsewhere and you are still unsatisfied. If
they are desires of the senses, immediately they are
satisfied you desire them again. The craver of
sexual excitement is not contented with last year's
or even yesterday's pleasures. The craving is without end. It is insatiable. Desirelessness brings liberty
and freedom, non-attachment is equanimity and
bliss.

Hatha Yoga prepares the body and mind for the
spiritual exercises of Raja Yoga. No other system so
perfectly and effectively realizes the ideal of *mens
sana in corpore sano*. Yoga shows the way to physical
and mental well-being. It integrates. It promotes a
balanced personality. It puts the whole being into
harmony with the universe. (It is interesting to note
that the Peckham experimenters defined health as
"wholeness".)

When a person has practised Yoga for some time
friends notice a great change in him. He looks and is,
healthier, brighter of eye, and clearer of skin. He is
more composed, relaxed, courteous, tactful, humble
and tolerant. He has control of his emotions, and
because of his self-mastery commands the respect of
others. He is at peace with himself and with the
universe.

In conclusion, let me point out that, as with other

practices, results are proportionate to the amount of effort expended.

As the *Hatha Yoga Pradipika* says:

"Whether young, old or too old, sick or lean, one who discards laziness, gets success if he practises Yoga. Success comes to him who is engaged in the practice; for by merely reading books on Yoga, one can never get success. Success cannot be attained by adopting a particular dress. It cannot be gained by telling tales. Practice alone is the means of success."

MEDITATION EXERCISES

Having seated yourself comfortably, select a quotation, concentrate quietly on its words and their meanings, think about it, ponder its truth. Ask yourself questions about it. What is the writer trying to say? Do you feel that what he says is true? What can you learn from it, and how can you apply it to enrich and develop your own spiritual life? Go on in this way until you have distilled the essence of the selected quotation. Then make a Samyama on that essence.

Whatever may be the charm of emotion, I do not know whether it equals the sweetness of those hours of silent meditation, in which we have a glimpse and foretaste of the contemplative joys of Paradise. Desire and fear, sadness and care, are done away. Existence is reduced to the simplest form, the most ethereal mode of being, that is, to pure self-consciousness. It is a state of harmony without tension and without disturbance, the dominical state of the soul, perhaps the state which awaits it beyond the grave. It is happiness as the Orientals understand it, the happiness of the anchorite, who neither struggles nor wishes any more, but simply adores and enjoys. It is difficult to find words in which to express this moral situation, for our languages can only render the

particular and localized vibrations of life; they are
incapable of expressing this motionless concentration,
this divine quietude, this state of the resting ocean,
which reflects the sky, and is master of its own pro-
fundities. Things are then re-absorbed into their
principles; memories are swallowed up in memory;
the soul is only soul, and is no longer conscious of
itself in its individuality and separateness. It is something which feels the universal life, a sensible atom of
the Divine, of God. It no longer appropriates anything
to itself, it is conscious of no void. Only the Yoghis
and Soufis perhaps have known in its profundity this
humble and yet voluptuous state, which combines
the joys of being and of non-being, which is neither
reflection nor will, which is above both the moral
existence and the intellectual existence, which is the
return to unity, to the pleroma, the vision of Plotinus
and of Proclus—Nirvana in its most attractive form.

AMIEL from his *Journal*

One who is at peace and is quiet no sorrow or harm
can enter, no evil breath can invade. Therefore, his
inner power remains whole and his spirit intact. . . .

Truly is it said, "If the bodily frame of a man labours
and has no rest, it wears itself out; if his spiritual
essence is used without cessation, then it flags, and
having flagged, runs dry.

"The nature of water is that if nothing is mixed with
it, it remains clear; if nothing ruffles it, it remains
smooth. But if it is obstructed so that it does not flow,

then too it loses its clearness. In these ways it is a symbol of the heavenly powers that are in man."

Truly is it said, "A purity unspoiled by any contamination, a peace and unity not disturbed by any variation, detachment and inactivity broken only by such movement as is in accord with the motions of Heaven —such are the secrets that conserve the soul."

CHUANG TZU (translated Waley).

The individual seeking for the law of his being can only find it safely if he regards clearly two great psychological truths and lives in that clear vision. First, the ego is not the self; there is one self of all and the soul is a portion of that universal Divinity. The fulfilment of the individual is not the utmost development of his egotistic intellect, vital force, physical well-being, and the utmost satisfaction of his mental, emotional, physical cravings, but the flowering of the divine in him to its utmost capacity of wisdom, power, love and universality, and through this flowering his utmost realization of all the possible beauty and delight of existence. . . .

The second psychic truth the individual has to grasp is this: that he is not only himself, but is in solidarity with all of his kind—let us leave aside for the moment that which seems to be not of his kind. That which we are has expressed itself through the individual, but also through the universality; and though each has to fulfil itself in its own way, neither can succeed independently of the other. . . .

This is what a true subjectivism teaches us—first, that we are a higher self than our ego or our members, secondly, that we are in our life and being not only ourselves but all others; for there is a secret solidarity which our egoism may kick at and strive against, but from which we cannot escape. It is the old Indian discovery that our real "I" is a Supreme Being which is our true self and which it is our business to discover and consciously become; and, secondly, that our Being is one in all, expressed in the individual and in the collectivity—and only by admitting and realizing our unity with others can we entirely fulfil our true self-being.   AUROBINDO. From *The Human Cycle*.

And this immortal and perfect soul must be the same in the highest God as well as in the humblest man, the difference between them being only in the degree in which this soul manifests itself.

VIVEKANANDA

Better keep yourself clean and bright: you are the window through which you must see the world.
GEORGE BERNARD SHAW. From
Man & Superman

Thou art man and woman, boy and girl; old and worn thou walkest bent over a staff; thou art the blue bird and the green and the scarlet-eyed.
From the *Swetaswatara Upanishad*

Wretched is the soul that does not feel its own

fruitfulness, and know itself to be big with life and love, as a tree with blossom in the spring!

ROMAIN ROLLAND. From *Jean-Christophe*

"The Sufi," says Jalal-uddin Rumi, "is the son of time present." Spiritual progress is a spiral advance. We start as infants in the animal eternity of life in the moment, without anxiety for the future or regret of the past; we grow up into the specifically human condition of those who look before and after, who live to a great extent, not in the present but in memory and anticipation, not spontaneously but by rule and with prudence, in repentance and fear and hope; and we can continue, if we so desire, up and on in a returning sweep towards a point corresponding to our starting place in animality, but incommensurably above it. Once more life is lived in the moment— the life now, not of a sub-human creature, but of a being in whom charity has cast out fear, vision has taken the place of hope, selflessness has put a stop to the positive egotism of complacent reminiscence and the negative egotism of remorse. The present moment is the only aperture through which the soul can pass out of time into eternity, through which grace can pass out of eternity into the soul, and through which charity can pass from one soul in time into another. That is why the Sufi and, along with him, every other practising exponent of the Perennial Philosophy is, or tries to be, a son of time present.

ALDOUS HUXLEY. From *The Perennial Philosophy*

It is eternity now. I am in the midst of it. It is about me in the sunshine; I am in it, as the butterfly floats in the light-laden air. Nothing has to come; it is now. Now is eternity; now is the immortal life. Here this moment, by this tumulus, on earth now; I exist in it. The years, the centuries, the cycles are absolutely nothing; it is only a moment since this tumulus was raised; in a thousand years more it will still be only a moment. To the soul there is no past and no future; all is and will be ever, in now.

RICHARD JEFFERIES. From *The Story of my Heart*

As a mother, even at the risk of her own life, protects her son, her only son, so let there be good will without measure between all beings. Let good will without measure prevail in the whole world, above, below, around, unstinted, unmixed with any feeling of differing or opposing interests. If a man remain steadfastly in this state of mind all the time he is awake, then is come to pass the saying, "Even in this world holiness has been found." *Metta Sutta*

By reason of the quite universal idea ... of participation in a common nature, it (thought) is compelled to declare the unity of mankind with all created beings.

ALBERT SCHWEITZER. From *Indian Thought and its Development*

The important thing is that we are part of life. We are born of other lives; we possess the capacities to bring still other lives into existence. In the same way, if we look into a microscope we see cell producing cell. . . . In the very fibres of our being, we bear within ourselves the fact of the solidarity of life.

ALBERT SCHWEITZER. From *The Ethics of Reverence for Life*

Of one tree are ye all the fruit and of one bough the leaves . . . The world is but one country and mankind its citizens . . . Let not a man glory in that he loves his country; let him rather glory in this, that he loves his kind. Sayings of BAHAULLAH.

He that saith he is in the light, and hateth his brother, is in darkness even until now.

He that loveth his brother abideth in the light, and there is none occasion of stumbling in him.

1 *John* 2, 9-10.

The whole length and breadth of the wide world is pervaded by the radiant thoughts of a mind all-embracing, vast and boundless, in which dwells no hate nor ill-will.

With radiant thoughts of love, of compassion, of sympathy and of poise his mind pervades each of the worlds four quarters above, below, across, everywhere.

From the *Vatthupuma Sutta*

What is love? To love mankind.

What is wisdom? To know mankind.

Saying of CONFUCIUS.

Though I speak with the tongues of men and of angels, and have not charity, I am become as sounding brass, or a tinkling cymbal.

And though I have the gift of prophecy, and understand all mysteries, and all knowledge; and though I have all faith, so that I could remove mountains, and have not charity, I am nothing.

And though I bestow all my goods to feed the poor, and though I give my body to be burned, and have not charity, it profiteth me nothing.

Charity suffereth long, and is kind; charity envieth not; charity vaunteth not itself, is not puffed up.

Doth not behave itself unseemly, seeketh not her own, is not easily provoked, thinketh no evil;

Rejoiceth not in iniquity, but rejoiceth in the truth;

Beareth all things, believeth all things, hopeth all things, endureth all things.

Charity never faileth: but whether there be prophecies, they shall fail; whether there be tongues, they shall cease; whether there be knowledge, it shall vanish away.

For we know in part, and we prophesy in part.

But when that which is perfect is come, then that which is in part shall be done away.

When I was a child, I spake as a child, I understood as a child, I thought as a child; but when I became a man, I put away childish things.

For now we see through a glass, darkly; but then face to face: now I know in part; but then shall I know even as also I am known.

And now abideth faith, hope, charity, these three; but the greatest of these is charity.

1 *Corinthians* 13.

What is it that makes atoms come and join atoms, molecule molecules, sets big planets flying towards each other, attracts man to woman, woman to man, human beings to human beings, animals to animals, drawing the whole universe, as it were, towards one centre? That is what is called love. Its manifestation is from the lowest atom to the highest ideal: omnipresent, all-pervading, everywhere is this love. . . . It is the one motive power that is in the universe. Under the impetus of that love, Christ stands to give up His life for humanity, Buddha for an animal, the mother for the child, the husband for the wife. It is under the impetus of the same love that men are ready to give up their lives for their country, and strange to say, under the impetus of that same love, the thief goes to steal, the murderer to murder; for in these cases, the spirit is the same. . . . The thief has love of gold, the love was there but it was misdirected. So, in all crimes, as well as in all virtuous actions, behind stands that eternal love. . . . The motive power of the universe is love, without which the universe will fall to pieces in a moment, and this love is God.

VIVEKANANDA. From *Bhakti Yoga*

Realize that thou art 'That'—Brahman which is supreme, beyond the range of all speech, but which may be known through the eye of pure wisdom. It is pure, absolute consciousness, the eternal substance.

The wise man in Samadhi perceives in his heart That something which is eternal Knowledge, pure Bliss, incomparable, eternally free, actionless, as limitless as space, stainless, without distinction of subject and object, and which is all-pervading Brahman (in essence).

SRI SANKARACHARYA. From *The Crest Jewel of Wisdom*. Verses 256 and 409.

The wise man severs quickly and completely, by means of the sword of Knowledge, the shackles created by conscious or unconscious action and dwells in the pure self. As a vast, roaring fire consumes wood, both dry and wet, so the fire of Knowledge destroys, in a moment, all good and evil actions. As a lotus leaf is not contaminated by water, though floating on it, so the knower of the Self is not contaminated by sound, touch, taste, etc. As a snake-charmer possessing the mantra power is not bitten by snakes, though playing with them, so the knower of the Self is not injured by the snakes of the sense-organs, though playing with them. As poison which has been swallowed by a man is digested through the power of mantra and medicine, so the sins of the wise are consumed instantaneously through the power of Knowledge.

From the *Sivadharmottara*

Unity is the touchstone of truth. All that contributes to unity is truth.

VIVEKANANDA. From *Practical Vedanta*

Peace is not lack of war, but an inner virtue, which has its source in the courage of the soul.

SPINOZA.

May all beings be happy and at their ease! May they be joyous and live in safety! All beings—whether weak or strong—omitting none—in high, middle, or low realms of existence, small or great, visible or invisible, near or far away, born or to be born—may all beings be happy and at their ease! Let none deceive another, or despise any being in any state; let none by anger or ill-will wish harm to another! Even as a mother watches over and protects her child, her only child, so with a boundless mind should one cherish all living beings, radiating friendliness over the entire world, above, below, and all around without limit; so let him cultivate a boundless goodwill towards the entire world, uncramped, free from ill-will or enmity.

From the *Metta Sutta*

May peace reign in the heavenly region, may it reign in the atmosphere, may it fill the four corners of the earth, may the waters be soothing and the medicinal herbs be healing; may plants be the source of peace to all creatures; may all enlightened persons bring peace to us; may the Vedas spread peace throughout; may all other objects everywhere give us peace, and may peace itself bring peace to all and may that peace come to me and remain with me forever.

OM
PEACE: PEACE: PEACE

Peace chant from the *Yajur-Veda*

GLOSSARY

Ahimsa . . .	Non-violence
Ajna	Command Chakra
Akasha . . .	Ether
Anahata . . .	Unstruck Sound Chakra
Apana	Outgoing breath
Aparigrapha . .	Non-receiving
Ardha-Matsyendrasana .	Twist Posture
Asanas . . .	Postures
Asteya	Non-stealing
Atman	The Individual Soul
Baddha Padmasana	Adept Posture
Basti . . .	One of the six purification practices
Bhakti Yoga . .	Union by love
Bhastrika . .	Bellows Breath
Bhujangasana .	Cobra Posture
Brahman . . .	The Overself; the Supreme Reality
Chakra . . .	Centre
Chakrasana . .	Wheel Posture
Chitta	Mind stuff
Dhanurasana .	Bow Posture
Dharana . . .	Concentration
Dhauti	One of the six purification practices
Dhyana . . .	Contemplation

Guru . . . . Yoga master

Halasana . . . Plough Posture
Hansah . . . I am He
Hatha Yoga . . . Union by bodily control

Ida . . . . Left nostril
Ishvara Pranidhana . Worship

Jalandhara . . . Chin-lock
Janusirasana . . . Knee and Head Posture
Japa . . . . Repetition of sacred syllables, words and mantras
Jnana Yoga . . . Union by knowledge

Kaivalya . . . Isolation
Kapalabhati . . . Cleansing Breath
Kukkutasana . . . Cock Posture
Kumbhaka . . . Breath suspension
Kundalini . . . Latent energy; 'The coiled serpent'

Manipura . . . Jewel City Chakra
Mantra Yoga . . Union by speech
Mantras . . . Prayers
Matsyasana . . . Fish Posture
Mayurasana . . . Peacock Posture
Muladhara . . . Root Chakra
Muni . . . . Sage

Nadas . . . . Mystic sounds
Nadis . . . . Nerves
Nauli . . . . One of the six purification practices

Neti	One of the six purification practices
Niyamas . . .	Observances
Om (Aum) . . .	Sacred syllable; symbol of Atman and Brahman; the basis of all sound
Padhahasthasana . .	Standing Posterior Stretch Posture
Padmasana . . .	Lotus Posture
Parbatasana . . .	Mountain Posture
Paschimatanasana .	Posterior Stretch Posture
Patanjali . . .	'The father of Yoga'
Pingala . . .	Right nostril
Prana . . .	The life force; incoming breath
Pranayama . . .	Breath control
Pratyahara . . .	Sense withdrawal
Puraka . . .	Inhalation
Purusha . . .	The inner Self
Sahasrara . . .	Thousand Petaled Lotus Chakra
Salabhasana . . .	Locust Posture
Samadhi . . .	Self-realization; Superconsciousness; the highest stage of Yoga practice
Samprajanya . .	Awareness
Samyama . .	The last three limbs of Yoga practised together
Santosha . . .	Contentment

Sarvangasana	. .	Shoulder Stand Posture
Satya . .	. .	Truthfulness
Shat Karma .	. .	The Purification Practices
Siddhas .	. .	Adepts
Siddhasana .	. .	Perfect Posture
Siddhis .	. .	Supra-natural powers
Sirsasana .	. .	Inverted Body Posture; Yoga Head Stand
Sitali . .	. .	A breathing exercise
Sitkari .	. .	A breathing exercise
Soham .	. .	He is I
Sukhasana .	. .	Easy Posture
Sukh Purvak .	. .	Comfortable Pranayama
Sunya . .	. .	The void
Supta-Vajrasana	. .	Pelvic Posture
Svadhishthana	. .	Support of Life Breath Chakra
Svadhyaya .	. .	Study
Syadvada .	. .	Philosophic doctrine resembling relativism
Tapa . .	. .	Austerity
Trataka .	. .	One of the six purification practices
Uddiyana .	. .	Retraction of the abdominal muscles
Ujjayi .	. .	Audible Breath
Uttanakurmakasana	.	Tortoise Posture
Vairagya .	. .	Detachment
Vishuddha .	. .	Great Purity Chakra
Vrittis .	. .	Thought waves

Yoga . . . . Union; 'to yoke'; merging of the individual with the universal soul

Yoga Mudra . . Symbol of Yoga Posture

RECOMMENDED READING

Aurobindo, Sri *Basis of Yoga* (Sri Aurobindo Ashram, Pondicherry. British stockists: Luzac & Co. Ltd)

Behanan, Kovoor T. *Yoga: A Scientific Evaluation* (Martin Secker and Warburg, Ltd.)

Bernard, Theos *Hatha Yoga* (Rider and Co., Ltd.) *Heaven Lies Within us* (Rider and Co., Ltd.)

Brunton, Paul *The Quest of the Overself* (Rider and Co., Ltd.) *The Wisdom of the Overself* (Rider and Co., Ltd.)

Danielou, Alain *Yoga: The Method of Re-Integration* (Christopher Johnson)

Evans-Wentz, W. Y., ed. *The Tibetan Book of the Dead* (Oxford University Press)

Huxley, Aldous *The Perennial Philosophy* (Chatto and Windus, Ltd.)

Kuvalayananda *Srimat Asanas* (Kaivalyadhama, Lonavla, Bombay) *Pranayama* (Kaivalyadhama, Lonavla, Bombay)

Muzumdar, S. *Yogic Exercises* (Orient Longmans, Ltd.)

Nicoll, Dr. Maurice *Living Time and the Integration of the Life* (Vincent Stuart Publishers, Ltd.)

Rele, V. G. *The Mysterious Kundalini* (D. B. Taraporevala Sons and Co., Bombay). *Yogic Asanas* (D. B. Taraporevala Sons and Co., Bombay)

Rolland, Romain *Prophets of the New India* (Cassell and Co., Ltd.)

Sadhu, Muni *In Days of Great Peace* (George Allen and Unwin, Ltd.)

Sinh, Pancham, tr. *Hatha Yoga Pradapika* (Lalit Mohan Basu, Allahabad)

Vithaldas, Yogi *The Yoga System of Health* (Faber and Faber, Ltd.)

Vivekananda, Swami *Raja-Yoga, or Conquering the Internal Nature* (Advaita Ashrama, Calcutta; Kegan Paul, Trench, Trubner & Co.); contains translation and commentary on Patanjali's *Yoga Sutras*

Wood, Prof. Ernest E. *Practical Yoga* (Rider and Co., Ltd.): a modern translation and commentary on Patanjali's *Yoga Sutras. Great Systems of Yoga* (Philosophical Library, New York)

Yesudian, Selvarajan and Haich, Elizabeth *Yoga and Health* (George Allen and Unwin, Ltd.) *Yoga: Uniting East and West* (George Allen and Unwin, Ltd.)

Yogendra, Shri *Yoga Personal Hygiene* (Yoga Institute, Bombay)

INDEX

Karate

—self defence or sport?
Exercise or philosophy?

The majority of its devotees are attracted by the self-defence movements on which it is based and there can be no doubt that it is the most effective form of self-defence. Karate is, however, far more than just this. It is an exercise in physical and mental balance and one of the toughest forms of physical training in existence. It is also claimed that it moulds the personality of its exponents.

OTHER BESTSELLING TITLES
IN THIS SERIES:

☐ 10902 5 **ORIGAMI** 25p

☐ 15071 8 **COMPUTER PROGRAMMING** 30p

☐ 14813 6 **KARATE** 30p

☐ 15072 6 **JUDO** 30p

☐ 14812 8 **INVESTMENT** 30p

HODDER PAPERBACKS, Cash Sales Department, Kernick Industrial Estate, Penryn, Cornwall.

Please send cheque or postal order. No currency, and allow 5p per book (4p per book on orders of 5 copies and over) to cover the cost of postage and packing in U.K., 5p per copy overseas.

Name..

Address ....

....

....